D0191409

ADVANCE PRAISE FOR

A Parkinson's Primer

Morton Kondracke: "John Vine has written the best primer I've ever read for newly diagnosed Parkinson's patients and their families. It helps them cope with the shock of diagnosis, gives them (jargon-free) the scientific basics they need to know, describes the symptoms they may experience (making clear that every case is different), and catalogs the resources available to navigate living with Parkinson's. John humanizes the book by describing his own experience and that of 22 other patients and their partners. I'd urge every neurologist to have copies of Vine's primer on hand to help new PD patients on their journey forward."

Morton Kondracke is the author of *Saving Milly: Love, Politics, and Parkinson's Disease* and a member of the Founders' Council of the Michael J. Fox Foundation.

Lesley Stahl: "My husband has PD, and I devoured this book. It's wise, wonderfully readable, and, above all, helpful. Since John Vine has PD, he speaks with great authority about the challenges, both physical and psychological. If you have Parkinson's, live with someone who has it, or just know someone battling the disease, *A Parkinson's Primer* is for you."

Lesley Stahl is an award-winning television journalist who regularly appears on the CBS News program *60 Minutes.*

Stephen Grill, MD, PhD: "This is a remarkable book describing the personal experiences of many individuals, including the author, living with Parkinson's disease. It captures the fact that although there are many possible symptoms in this disease, each person experiences different symptoms and copes with them in various ways. The thoughtful and insightful comments and coping strategies should be helpful for persons with PD, and their partners, regardless of the stage of the disease."

Stephen Grill is Director of the Parkinson's & Movement Disorders Center of Maryland.

A Parkinson's
PRIMER

*An Indispensable Guide
to Parkinson's Disease
for Patients and Their Families*

JOHN M. VINE

PAUL DRY BOOKS

Philadelphia 2017

Caution
This book does not provide medical or legal advice.
If you want medical advice, please consult a physician.
If you want legal advice, please consult a lawyer.

First Paul Dry Books Edition, 2017

Paul Dry Books, Inc.
Philadelphia, Pennsylvania
www.pauldrybooks.com

Copyright © 2017 John M. Vine

All rights reserved

Printed in the United States of America

Library of Congress Cataloging-in-Publication Data

Names: Vine, John M., author.
Title: A Parkinson's primer : an indispensable guide to Parkinson's disease
   for patients and their families / John M. Vine.
Description: Philadelphia : Paul Dry Books, 2017. | Includes bibliographical
   references and index.
Identifiers: LCCN 2016049651 | ISBN 9781589881198 (paperback)
Subjects: LCSH: Vine, John M.,—Mental health. | Parkinson's disease—
   Patients—Biography. | Parkinson's disease—Patients—Family relationships. |
   BISAC: HEALTH & FITNESS / Diseases / Nervous System (incl. Brain). |
   HEALTH & FITNESS / Reference. | HEALTH & FITNESS / Diseases /
   General. | BIOGRAPHY & AUTOBIOGRAPHY / Personal Memoirs.
Classification: LCC RC382 .V56 2017 | DDC 616.8/330092 [B] —dc23
LC record available at https://lccn.loc.gov/2016049651

To Joanne,
my partner in more ways than one

"Adversity introduces us to ourselves."

Author unknown, although similar
thoughts have been attributed to Einstein
and H. L. Mencken, among others

Preface

If you were recently diagnosed with Parkinson's disease ("Parkinson's" or "PD"), I hope you will read this book. I wrote it for you.

If you are a relative or friend of someone who was recently diagnosed with Parkinson's, I hope that you too will read this book. I wrote it for you as well.

I am a Parkinson's patient. I am not a physician or a scientist. I wrote this book to help Parkinson's patients become better patients, to help their relatives become better relatives, and to help their friends become better friends.

When I was diagnosed with Parkinson's, I was 60 years old, average for a newly diagnosed Parkinson's patient. I was shocked by the news. I did not know what Parkinson's was. As far as I knew, no member of my family had been diagnosed with the disease. I had no history of neurological problems. I thought I was basically healthy, as did my wife, Joanne.

Joanne and I were overwhelmed at first. The literature on Parkinson's was voluminous. It offered more information than we could absorb at that time. We needed a primer that was written from a recently diagnosed patient's perspective.

This is the book that Joanne and I needed. It is designed to get the patient—and the patient's family and friends—started.

I have tried to express myself plainly. As much as possible, I have avoided using Greek- and Latin-based medical terms, and when I could not avoid using them, I have tried to make their meaning clear.

In Appendix 1, I address some of the myths and misconceptions about Parkinson's disease. For example, Parkinson's is sometimes referred to as a "movement disorder," and Parkinson's specialists are sometimes called "movement disorders specialists." However, Parkinson's has numerous *nonmovement* symptoms, and I have tried, throughout the book, to clear up any confusion caused by references to movement symptoms.

Similarly, Parkinson's is sometimes referred to as a "disorder of the brain" despite mounting evidence that it is *not* exclusively a brain disease. Because I am concerned that "brain disorder" terminology could also be confusing, I have tried throughout the book to make clear that Parkinson's might not be exclusively a brain disease.

I do not refer to people with Parkinson's as "victims" as some commentators do. Calling people "victims" implies that they have no control over their condition. In fact, people with Parkinson's *can* influence the course of the disease. I prefer to use the term "patients." Victims commiserate about their misfortunes. Patients get treatment.

Likewise, I do not use the term "caregiver" to refer to the people who care for Parkinson's patients. "Caregiver" implies that Parkinson's patients are merely "care receivers." This is far from the truth. Most Parkinson's patients are largely responsible for their own care, especially in the years immediately following their diagnosis. Accordingly, I refer to the people who care for Parkinson's patients as the patients' "partners."

When I started to work on this book, I knew how Parkinson's was affecting my own life, but I had only a very general idea of how it affects others. One of my first steps, then, was to begin interviewing a wide range of patients and their partners. This book is based in large part on those interviews. Stories and quotations from the interviewees are featured throughout the text. A list of the interviewees is provided in Appendix 2.

My interviews of Parkinson's patients and their partners have only increased my regard and affection for them. All received me warmly. All were eager to be helpful and generous with their time and their thoughts. All were candid—even when being candid was not easy. All conducted themselves with dignity and without self-pity. They inspired me to deal with Parkinson's in a like manner.

This book is also the result of the efforts of many others, including neurologists and other physicians, scientists, therapists, friends and family members, and other members of the Parkinson's community. I am grateful for their generous and thoughtful contributions, as detailed in the Acknowledgments section at the end of the book.

This "Primer," as I have called it, covers only the basics about Parkinson's. I encourage those who wish to learn more to consult other sources. The organizations and publications identified in Appendix 3 and the Bibliography are good places to start. The patient's neurologist might have recommendations as well.

John M. Vine
Washington, DC

Contents

CHAPTER 1

Diagnosis

Symptoms

PARKINSON'S CREPT UP on me. The early symptoms of the disease were so subtle and progressed so slowly that it was remarkably easy for me to dismiss them as signs of advancing age.

I turned 60 in 2004. I felt healthy. Thanks to successful surgery, prostate cancer—the only serious medical problem I had encountered in my adult life—was four years behind me. I looked forward to completing my career at the law firm in Washington, DC, where I had practiced law since 1971. I also looked forward to retirement years that would give me more time to devote to my wife and family and to the travel, writing, photography, and other hobbies that I had largely neglected while practicing law.

True, in recent years my handwriting—which had never been good—had deteriorated significantly. I often could not read my own notes. I had greater difficulty with a keyboard. My hands and arms ached after only a few minutes of typing, and my typing errors mounted. I thought I might have carpal tunnel syndrome, but nothing more serious than that.

Oh, yes, there was also that nettlesome tremor in my right arm. It was particularly noticeable when I went outside in the morning to collect our daily newspaper. The tremor, I thought, was probably just a symptom of aging. I blew it off. I told myself that my father (who lived until his 90s) also had a very minor tremor in one of his hands in his later years, and so did one of my brothers (15 months younger than I). Nothing serious, I told myself.

One other thing. I was a little unsteady when I went downstairs to have breakfast each morning. No big deal. I didn't fall. I didn't even come close to falling. Nothing I couldn't accommodate by holding on to the railing.

Other members of my family were not so sure. Joanne, my wife, was particularly concerned about the tremor in my right arm. "You really should have that looked at," she advised me.

Finally, I scheduled what I expected to be a routine office visit with my internist. Joanne reminded me, once again, to ask him about the tremor. I did not believe it was necessary to do so, but I also believed it would be foolish to ignore my wife.

I had first met my internist in 1963, when we were students at Amherst College. In 2004 he had been my physician for more than 30 years. It took him about five minutes to reach a tentative conclusion. He told me that because of our personal relationship, he would be more direct with me than with most other patients: "I think you have Parkinson's disease," he said. I knew that Muhammad Ali (the activist and former boxing champ), Michael J. Fox (the actor), and Janet Reno (the former U.S. attorney general) had this disease. Beyond that, I didn't know what Parkinson's was. I knew (or thought I knew) it wasn't good, but not much more than that.

Oddly, I did not feel emotional. I was curious about what would follow from the diagnosis, but for reasons I cannot explain, I felt calm and dispassionate. It was almost as though my internist and I were talking about another patient.

My internist instructed me to see a particular neurologist with considerable experience in caring for Parkinson's patients. He emphasized that I should see this particular doctor, not just any neurologist. But scheduling an appointment in the near future with the neurologist required considerable patience and persistence. At last, after my internist intervened and spoke directly to the neurologist, I was able to make an appointment.

Joanne accompanied me to the neurologist's office. She wanted to hear, first-hand, what he had to say. After examining me, he told us that my internist was probably correct, that I probably had Parkinson's, but that he wanted to rule out other possibilities, such as a brain tumor. We made arrangements for a magnetic resonance imaging (MRI) scan. An MRI machine uses a magnetic field and radio waves to create detailed images of structures inside the body. In the early stages of Parkinson's disease, an MRI scan of the brain usually appears normal. Although an MRI is usually not necessary, the neurologist used the MRI to make sure there was no other reason for my symptoms.

After the MRI results were analyzed, Joanne and I returned to the neurologist. He smiled. "I have good news for you," he said. "At least, I hope you'll consider it good news. You have Parkinson's."

The Basics of Parkinson's

Although it might seem absurd to call a Parkinson's diagnosis "good news," I thought I understood what the neurologist meant. Compared with some other possibilities, such as a brain tumor, Parkinson's was less alarming.

The neurologist told me that Parkinson's was not necessarily fatal or debilitating, that it was treatable, that an informed patient could influence the therapy he or she received, and that most people who were diagnosed with Parkinson's could remain active and productive for many years. If she were still alive and heard the neurologist's report, my great-grandmother might have said, "It could be worse."

Indeed, some of the alternatives *were* much worse. Not long after I was diagnosed, I called a contemporary of mine at another Washington law firm to discuss an article I had written. Although we had known each other for nearly 30 years, we were not close friends and had not spoken in several years. When he got on the telephone, he mumbled. I could barely understand him. I told him he sounded like he had just returned from a visit to the dentist. I straightened up when he said it was a medical rather than a dental problem.

"I hope it isn't serious," I said.

"I'm afraid it is," he replied.

He had amyotrophic lateral sclerosis, often referred to as ALS or Lou Gehrig's disease. He died not long after our call.

So some of the alternatives were worse. But that was only part of the neurologist's message. My prospects for living a fulfilling and active life with Parkinson's were much better than I recognized.

Chris Whitmer: "There are worse things than having Parkinson's. My mother had ALS, and she died within a year. At least I can watch my kids grow up."

Parkinson's is the second most prevalent neurodegenerative disease in the United States. Only Alzheimer's outranks it. Approximately 60,000 people are diagnosed with Parkinson's each year in the United States. The total number of people who have Parkinson's is uncertain, but some estimates run as high as a million or more in the United States alone. For a variety of reasons, many people with Parkinson's are never diagnosed by a physician as having the disease. Some people simply don't consult a physician. Others consult a physician but don't receive the correct diagnosis.

An accurate diagnosis is critical. To receive an accurate diagnosis, many patients consult a movement disorders specialist, a neurologist who has received additional training in Parkinson's and other movement disorders. Experts have found that a Parkinson's diagnosis by a movement disorders specialist is correct 98.6% of the time.

Other patients consult a general neurologist, a neurologist who may treat patients with any of over 100 neurological conditions. In some cases, Parkinson's can be difficult for some non-specialists to diagnose, however. Many people who are ultimately considered to have Parkinson's were previously told by a general neurologist that they did *not* have Parkinson's. A surprisingly high percentage (perhaps 25%) of those initially diagnosed with

Parkinson's by a general neurologist are later told that they do not have the disease.

What can make Parkinson's difficult for a nonspecialist to diagnose is the fact that most Parkinson's cases (approximately 90%) are sporadic. In medical terminology, "sporadic" does not mean intermittent; rather, it means that the disease occurs randomly, with no known cause. There is currently no blood test or other laboratory test that can be used to diagnose sporadic Parkinson's. As a result, the determination that a patient has Parkinson's is usually based on the patient's medical history and a neurologist's evaluation of the patient's symptoms. Neurologists sometimes also use tests to exclude the possibility that some other disorder is responsible for the patient's symptoms. Usually, however, a diagnosis can be made without any testing.

Obtaining treatment for Parkinson's requires the patient to make numerous visits to the doctor. A knowledgeable and experienced doctor and an open and comfortable relationship between patient and doctor are prerequisites for good care. If a patient has difficulty identifying an appropriate neurologist, the patient should ask his or her primary care doctor for a referral. If the patient belongs to a support group, the patient also might seek recommendations from other members of the group.

In 1913 a pathologist by the name of Frederick Lewy observed that the brain cells of deceased Parkinson's patients contained microscopic clumps of protein, now known as Lewy bodies. Even today, Lewy bodies can be detected only during an autopsy. According to a National Institutes of Health (NIH) report, autopsies have uncovered Lewy bodies in the brains of many older persons who had not been diagnosed with Parkinson's. One study found Lewy bodies in 8% of people over 50, in almost 13% of people over 70, and in almost 16% of those over 80. As a result, some experts call Parkinson's an "iceberg phenomenon," lurking undetected in many older people who show no outward signs of the disease.

The literature on Parkinson's disease is loaded with statistics of the sort I have been mentioning. Some of the basic statistics are presented in the accompanying table. The wide range of many of the numbers in the table suggests that these are no more than rough estimates. At the present time, there is no central repository where aggregate information about Parkinson's patients is collected.

In any event, statistics mask the wide variation in Parkinson's symptoms. Like some other diseases (multiple sclerosis, for ex-

Parkinson's Statistics

Category	Estimate	Source*
People with PD		
Total worldwide	7-10 million	Parkinson's Disease Foundation
Total in USA	500,000 to 1 million	Parkinson's Disease Foundation
Number diagnosed per year in USA	50,000-60,000	Parkinson's Disease Foundation; National Institute of Neurological Disorders and Stroke (NINDS), "Parkinson's Disease: Hope Through Research"
Undiagnosed	2 for each person diagnosed	Lieberman & McCall, *100 Questions & Answers About Parkinson Disease*, p. 4
Average age at onset	60	NINDS, "Parkinson's Disease: Hope Through Research"
Percentage of people age 60 and older with PD	1.5%-2.0%	Sweeney, "Parkinson's Disease"
Percentage of people age 80 or older with PD	2%	Palfreman, *Brain Storms*, p. 6
Percentage of PD patients under age 50	4%-15%	NINDS, "Parkinson's Disease: Hope Through Research"; Lieberman & McCall, p. 4; Parkinson's Disease Foundation
Percentage of PD patients age 40 or younger	As many as 10%	Lieberman & McCall, p. 4
Interval between onset and diagnosis	2-5 years or longer	Lieberman & McCall, p. 4

*For detailed citations of the sources mentioned here and elsewhere, see the Bibliography.

ample), Parkinson's has been called a "snowflake" disease. Just as no two snowflakes are identical, no two Parkinson's patients have identical symptoms. An individual Parkinson's patient does not necessarily have all or even most of the typical Parkinson's symptoms. Some symptoms show up in some patients but not in others; some symptoms appear sooner in some patients than in others; and some symptoms are more pronounced in some patients than in others. This is why, in writing this book, I have chosen to rely not only on my personal experience but also on the experiences of other Parkinson's patients and their partners.

· · ·

Early in 1989, Joel Havemann, then 45 years old, was introduced to Parkinson's at a business lunch in a restaurant. Joel ordered raspberries for dessert, but found it difficult to get the berries into his mouth. Joel's hand was shaky, and the fruit kept falling off his spoon. Within a few months, the tremors became more pronounced, and Joel's arm and leg muscles grew increasingly stiff and rigid. His posture deteriorated. Although Joel had a number of classic Parkinson's symptoms, the first neurologist he consulted concluded that he did not have Parkinson's. The neurologist offered three explanations for this conclusion.

The first was that an MRI had not shown any decay in the part of the brain where Parkinson's originates. In fact, an MRI lacks the power required to reveal the destruction of the nerve cells affected by Parkinson's.

The second explanation was that Joel's tremor was confined to Joel's right arm and leg, whereas Parkinson's generally involves both sides of the body. In fact, tremors and other Parkinson's movement symptoms generally begin on one side of the body and gradually expand to the other side.

The third explanation was that Parkinson's rarely applies to people as young as age 45. That is true but misleading. Although the average age of a newly diagnosed Parkinson's patient is 60, as many as 15% of Parkinson's patients are younger than 50, and as many as 10% are 40 or younger.

Dissatisfied with the advice he was getting, Joel consulted a neurologist who specialized in diagnosing Parkinson's in young people. This doctor promptly concluded that Joel had Parkinson's.

· · ·

Learie Phillip was introduced to Parkinson's in the front seat of his automobile after he had brought it to a stop at a busy intersection on New Hampshire Avenue in Maryland, just outside of Washington, DC. As Learie waited for a traffic light to turn green, his right foot was on the car's brake pedal. When the light changed, however, nothing happened. The car didn't move. No light, buzzer, or bell announced an automotive malfunction.

To the contrary, the problem was the driver. Learie tried to lift his right foot off the car's brake pedal and slide it over to the accelerator, but he could not do it. It was a routine step for an experienced driver. But on that day, in the year 2000, after more than 30 years of driving experience, Learie could not move his foot from the brake to the accelerator.

Learie received no sympathy from the drivers of the cars lined up behind him. They honked their horns impatiently as he struggled, without success, to lift his right foot. After what seemed like an eternity, Learie used his hands and arms to lift his right leg up, move the leg a bit to the right, and then place his foot on the accelerator. At last he felt relief—both because he had extricated himself from a very frustrating situation and because he realized that his predicament would have been far more serious if the car had been moving and he had been unable to move his foot from the accelerator to the brake.

At the time, Learie hoped that this was a bizarre but isolated episode. However, when it happened a second time, only a few minutes later, he was alarmed.

Learie's wife, Cecile, a dentist, urged him to consult a neurologist, and he promptly did so. The neurologist's diagnosis was immediate and unequivocal: Learie had Parkinson's.

• • •

Pete Riehm was introduced to Parkinson's in a podiatrist's office. Pete was seeing the doctor in order to get a second opinion regarding the consequences of a urinary tract infection.

Pete's primary care physician had treated the infection by prescribing the popular antibiotic Cipro, a drug that, according to the Food and Drug Administration (FDA), can increase the risk of tendinitis and tendon rupture in some patients. As it happened, several tendons in Pete's right ankle and foot ruptured soon after he took the Cipro, and Pete consulted one podiatrist and then another for advice.

Before he examined Pete's ankle and foot, the second podiatrist asked Pete whether he had Parkinson's. When Pete said he did not, the podiatrist asked whether he had ever been tested for the disease. When Pete said no, the podiatrist announced, "You will be tested now."

This podiatrist had noticed several tell-tale symptoms, including a tremor that Pete had developed only recently and poor muscle control in his right forearm. Two hours later Pete was seeing a neurologist, who did not take long to conclude that Pete had Parkinson's.

• • •

Cassandra Peters knew that something was wrong. She was depressed. She was uncharacteristically inactive and had little interest in anything or anyone. She also had a tremor. Since her father had been afflicted by a disorder called essential tremor, Cassandra thought that she had essential tremor too. Her doctors agreed. They attributed her lack of energy to menopause and depression.

Cassandra's symptoms advanced, however. She began dragging her left foot; her tremor began to spread; and her anxiety became more severe. Alarmed, Cassandra returned to the neurologist who had diagnosed her with essential tremor. This time, he concluded that she had Parkinson's. He told her to educate herself about the disease, but provided very little information and no guidance on what she should read.

After leaving the neurologist's office, Cassandra and her husband spent the rest of the day at a book store, browsing books on Parkinson's. By the end of the day, Cassandra was so frightened she was shaking. Her husband had to pick her up and carry her from the store to their car.

• • •

After Rick Vaughan was diagnosed with Parkinson's in 2008, he tried to figure out when he initially developed the disease. According to Rick, it was apparent in 2006 that his right-side motor skills, especially the fine motor skills in his right hand, were deteriorating. By then, Rick had begun to use his left hand to do what he had done in the past with his right (brushing his teeth and shaving, for example).

To trace the disease back earlier than 2006, Rick examined old photos taken of him. In some of them, he noticed, he was holding his right arm in a rigid way. On this basis he decided that his right-side symptoms began to emerge in 2003 or 2004, about five years before he was diagnosed with Parkinson's.

• • •

Glenn Roberts realized that he had Parkinson's before his doctors did. Glenn had only recently turned 50, and he did not have a tremor. Perhaps that is why Glenn's doctors, including his neurologist, initially missed the diagnosis.

Glenn did have a number of symptoms consistent with Parkinson's: lack of arm swing, deteriorating handwriting, and difficulty planting his feet on the ground when walking. So when Glenn read an article about Michael J. Fox in *Time Magazine*, he recognized the symptoms and consulted a prominent specialist, who promptly confirmed Glenn's self-diagnosis.

• • •

At least as far back as 2000, Scott Kragie developed sleep, concentration, and constipation problems. In order to address these problems, Scott saw a psychopharmacologist (a psychiatrist specializing in medication management) from 2002 until 2007. By

2007, however, it was apparent that the drugs prescribed by the psychopharmacologist were not working. Observing that Scott's lack of blinking and lack of facial expression suggested parkinsonism, the psychopharmacologist suggested that Scott consult his internist.

The internist thought that Scott might have Parkinson's and ordered an MRI to rule out a brain tumor. When the MRI indicated no tumor, the internist referred Scott to a neurologist. After examining Scott, however, the neurologist was uncertain about the diagnosis because Scott had no movement symptoms. "Time will tell," the doctor said.

Quite by chance, about six months later, Scott had dinner with an old friend, a cancer researcher by profession. The following day, the friend called Scott and said that he had noticed symptoms (including Scott's speech) that warranted further investigation. The friend suggested that Scott be evaluated at NIH, and Scott promptly arranged to have that done.

The doctors at NIH viewed Scott's case as unusual because his cognitive symptoms predominated over his movement symptoms. These doctors concluded that Scott probably did have a form of Parkinson's disease that they classified as "atypical Parkinson's."

A few weeks later, when Scott and his wife, Barbara, were out for a walk, they encountered a neighbor who happened to be a neurologist. After Scott described his condition, the neighbor explained that he was a movement disorders specialist and offered to examine Scott.

The neighbor was on the faculty of a nearby medical school and had focused on the nonmovement aspects of Parkinson's. After examining Scott, the neighbor showed him an article about Parkinson's nonmovement aspects and referred to mounting evidence that some of these symptoms (constipation and a diminished sense of smell, for example) may precede the emergence of Parkinson's classic movement features. The article described sleep, concentration, and constipation problems identical to Scott's symptoms. Scott's neurologist neighbor had no doubt that Scott had Parkinson's.

CHAPTER 2

Why Me?

In 2004 I considered myself a victim of bad luck. I had been diagnosed with Parkinson's disease. I had been told that Parkinson's was a brain disorder, that its cause was unknown, that it would gradually get worse, and that there was no known cure. I also had been told that the consequences of the disease were unpredictable but might include tremors, falling, impaired speech, hallucinations, delusions, dementia, and clinical depression.

Since the vast majority of 60-year-olds (98% or more) did not have this disease, I wondered why I had drawn the short straw. "Why *me*?" I asked myself. "What have I done to deserve this? Why did this insidious disease strike *me*?"

I soon recognized that there was no answer to the "Why me?" question and that, indeed, "Why me?" was the wrong question. I found it more productive to focus on what I now consider the right question: Why *not* me?

For some 60 years, I had lived a life blessed by good luck. I was raised by loving parents in a warm and nurturing environment; I was well educated; and I had enjoyed a successful professional career. I had an adoring (and adorable) wife and four loyal, supportive, and accomplished sons. Until recently I had enjoyed a life remarkably free of significant health problems.

It finally dawned on me that the "Why me?" question was based on the erroneous assumption that I was entitled to an illness-free life. I ultimately recognized that I had no such entitlement. I had no reason to believe that chronic illnesses were reserved exclusively for *other* people. In fact, few were better suited to having Parkinson's than I was. Few were better equipped to face the challenges that the disease presents.

I also recognized that I had been badly mistaken in viewing myself as a victim of bad luck. On the whole, my life had been blessed by *good* luck. True, Parkinson's had broken my streak of good luck, but it had not erased all of my previous good fortune. I resolved to try to make the best of the cards I had been dealt, and not to waste more time wondering why the cards had been dealt as they had.

Actually, as I later learned, I was *lucky* to have been diagnosed in 2004. The FDA had approved deep brain stimulation (DBS) surgery as a treatment for Parkinson's symptoms only two years earlier. In DBS surgery, now the most widely used form of surgery for Parkinson's, a neurosurgeon places two small electrodes in precise locations in the patient's brain. The surgeon then connects each electrode to a wire that runs from the electrode, under the patient's skin, to a battery-powered device, similar to a cardiac pacemaker, placed under the skin on the patient's chest wall. After the device is programmed, it is used to stimulate the particular brain cells targeted by the neurosurgeon.

I had DBS surgery in 2008. So far at least, it appears to have been a success. I now take less medication than I did before the surgery, and my symptoms have not advanced appreciably since then.

I do not feel helpless. I recognize that I have the power to manage my symptoms. I decide how to use that power. I don't have the power to make Parkinson's go away, but I do have the power to overcome some of the obstacles that Parkinson's creates.

Moreover, I am not alone. I have allies. Parkinson's has introduced me to many courageous, dedicated, and generous members of the Parkinson's community—patients and their partners, physicians, and therapists—whom I probably would not have met if I did not have the disease. Together with my family and friends, they have helped me enormously.

Parkinson's has opened more doors for me than it has closed. Although I now walk rather than run, I did not enjoy running in the first place. I walk more often, for longer periods of time, and for a purpose now; walking is part of my therapy. In addition, I am learning a lot about the disease, about other patients, about the human brain, and about myself.

Parkinson's has presented me with opportunities to enrich my life. Parkinson's has encouraged me to retire earlier than I otherwise would have, and I now take advantage of opportunities (for travel, writing, and photography, for example) that I had previously put on the back burner.

CHAPTER 3

Why Parkinson's?

Symptoms

IN 1817 a London physician named James Parkinson defined what is now called "Parkinson's disease" by describing the disease's symptoms: tremor, muscle rigidity, lack (or slowness) of movement, and balance and walking difficulties. Parkinson established the disease as a recognized medical condition. Today, two centuries later, although much more is known about the disease, its diagnosis is still based on Parkinson's description of its symptoms.

It is not possible to predict with confidence the symptoms that a Parkinson's patient will have or when those symptoms will emerge. Some symptoms are evident at the time the patient is diagnosed; others may not emerge until many years later; and still others may never emerge.

Some symptoms reinforce the consequences of other Parkinson's symptoms. For example, many Parkinson's symptoms—such as muscle rigidity, slowness of movement, balance problems, low blood pressure, fatigue, and impaired executive function—make it more difficult for the patient to walk and increase the risk of falling. Similarly, low blood pressure and the loss of deep sleep make it more likely that the patient will feel fatigued.

In addition, the side effects of some Parkinson's medications resemble some of the symptoms of the disease. As a result, it can be difficult to discern whether a particular symptom is caused by the disease, by the medication, or by both. For instance, impulsive behavior, low blood pressure, and sleeping problems may be caused by Parkinson's, by Parkinson's medications, or by both.

Parkinson's consequences can vary remarkably from patient to patient. For example, Parkinson's can cause some patients to be in motion and others to be motionless, some to be sleepy and others to be sleepless, some to have oily skin and others to have dry skin, and some to sweat excessively and some to sweat insufficiently.

Parkinson's is more prevalent among men than among women. Recent studies indicate, however, that while men may have more severe movement symptoms than do women, women may have more severe nonmovement symptoms than do men.

The Brain

Parkinson's is, at least in part, a disease of the human brain. The brain is the most complex part of the human body. In fact, the human brain is probably the most complex thing on Earth. The human brain is far more complex and powerful than the most advanced computer. Scientists are now only beginning to understand how the brain works.

Neurons. The primary unit of the brain is the brain cell or neuron. The brain consists of roughly three pounds of neurons floating in four to five ounces of fluid inside the skull. It is estimated that a normal human brain contains approximately 86 billion neurons. Whatever the precise number of neurons, that figure is large by almost any standard—much larger, in fact, than the number of people currently living on Earth (about 7.3 billion).

Neurotransmitters. Neurons send signals to other neurons by releasing (or secreting) chemicals called neurotransmitters. The brain uses neurotransmitters to instruct the heart to beat, the lungs to breathe, and the stomach to digest. Neurotransmitters can affect mood, sleep, and concentration. Current estimates are that the brain has more than 100 neurotransmitters, each with a specific function or functions.

Some neurotransmitters are excitatory; others are inhibitory; and still others are both excitatory and inhibitory. Excitatory neurotransmitters stimulate the brain. Inhibitory transmitters calm the brain and help create balance. Inhibitory neurotransmitters are easily depleted when excitatory neurotransmitters are overactive.

Neuronal networks. Neurons communicate with each other through highly structured neuronal networks. Each neuron receives signals from, and sends signals to, other neurons in complex brain circuits. It is estimated that one neuron can receive messages from, and send signals to, up to 10,000 other neurons. Neurons are separated from other neurons by small gaps, called synapses.

When a neurotransmitter is released by one neuron (call it "Neuron #1"), the neurotransmitter leaves what is called the axon terminal of Neuron #1, travels across a synapse to another neuron ("Neuron #2"), and attaches itself to a receptor on Neuron #2. An electrical signal is then activated or inhibited in Neuron #2. If the electrical signal reaches the end of Neuron #2, Neuron #2 itself releases a neurotransmitter, which travels across a synapse and attaches itself to yet another neuron. The cycle then begins again.

Parkinson's Effects on the Brain

Parkinson's disease reduces the levels of three of the brain's neurotransmitters: norepinephrine, serotonin, and dopamine.

Norepinephrine is an excitatory neurotransmitter. It is responsible for stimulatory processes in the body. It is the principal chemical messenger of the sympathetic nervous system, the part of the nervous system that controls many of the body's automatic body functions, such as pulse and blood pressure. Norepineph-rine also helps to control mental focus and emotional stability.

Serotonin is an inhibitory neurotransmitter; it does not stim-ulate the brain. It regulates appetite, sleep, memory, learning, mood, and muscle contraction, among other things. Adequate amounts of serotonin are required for a mood to be stable and to balance any excessive excitatory neurotransmitter firing in the brain.

Dopamine has both excitatory and inhibitory characteristics. Dopamine performs important functions in the regulation of body movements, memory, cognition, mental focus, sleep, moti-vation, and mood. A dopamine deficiency may cause the body's movements to become delayed and uncoordinated. By contrast, an excess of dopamine may cause the body to make unnecessary movements.

Parkinson's symptoms develop when approximately 60% to 80% of the dopamine in the brain has been depleted. The loss of dopamine interferes with the individual's ability to control his or her movements. In addition, a loss of dopamine may impair the brain's capacity to process and remember information and to concentrate. The loss of dopamine also may alter the individ-ual's mood.

Changes in the brain's neurochemistry resulting from declin-ing levels of norepinephrine, serotonin, and dopamine—together with the stress of a chronic disease—may help to explain why a significant percentage (perhaps 40% to 50%) of Parkinson's pa-tients experience clinical depression at some point during the course of the disease.

The substantia nigra. "Substantia nigra" is Latin for "dark sub-stance." The substantia nigra is a crescent-shaped, darkly pig-mented mass, located in the mid-brain region, at the top of the brain stem.

Neurons in the substantia nigra produce dopamine. Parkin-son's disease causes dopamine-producing neurons in the sub-stantia nigra to die. A dopamine deficiency in the substantia nigra leads to Parkinson's movement symptoms.

Lewy bodies. As I mentioned in Chapter 1, the brain cells of deceased Parkinson's patients contain microscopic clumps of protein, known as Lewy bodies. The Lewy bodies can be found in particular areas of deceased Parkinson's patients' brains, including the substantia nigra.

Alpha-synuclein. The primary component of a Lewy body is a protein called alpha-synuclein. Although alpha-synuclein's function in healthy cells is uncertain, there is considerable evidence suggesting that it plays a key role in the development of Parkinson's disease.

Ordinarily, alpha-synuclein readily dissolves in cell fluids. However, under certain conditions, it becomes insoluble and tends to aggregate and accumulate in clumps. The accumulation of the insoluble form of alpha-synuclein may compromise a cell's capacity to dispose of additional alpha-synuclein. The resulting build-up of alpha-synuclein may be toxic to brain cells and cause neuron dysfunction.

Alpha-synuclein pathology has also been discovered outside the body systems traditionally associated with Parkinson's, offering support for the emerging theory that Parkinson's affects many areas beyond the substantia nigra and extends beyond the central nervous system itself. In fact, Parkinson's earliest symptoms include constipation and other gastrointestinal problems. There is even evidence suggesting that Parkinson's appears in intestinal nerve cells *before* it appears in the brain.

What Causes Parkinson's?

The ultimate cause of Parkinson's disease is not known. There may be no single cause. Many scientists think that genetic defects combined with exposure to certain neurotoxins, such as pesticides or other chemicals, probably cause the disease. However, although various theories have been proposed for the cause of Parkinson's, no theory has been fully supported by hard facts. At this point, the best we can do is to list certain risk factors.

Researchers have identified a number of risk factors that appear to be correlated with the onset of Parkinson's:

- ***Pesticides and herbicides:*** There is evidence that implicates pesticides and herbicides as possible factors in some cases of Parkinson's.

- ***Rural areas:*** The risk of having Parkinson's is higher among people who live in rural areas than among others, and it is particularly high among agricultural workers and among people who drink private well water.

- ***Age:*** The risk of incurring Parkinson's is age-related. The peak age of onset of Parkinson's is 60 (my age at diagnosis). About 80% of Parkinson's patients develop Parkinson's between ages 40 and 70. As many as 10% of Parkinson's patients develop the disorder at or before age 40.

- ***Genetics:*** Specific genetic factors appear to account for early-onset Parkinson's, a relatively uncommon form of the disease that affects people diagnosed before age 50. If an individual has a parent or sibling who developed Parkinson's at a younger age, the individual has a higher than average risk of developing Parkinson's. However, if an individual has a relative who developed Parkinson's at an advanced age, the individual's risk of developing Parkinson's appears to be about average. Genetic testing is available for certain genes that have been linked to Parkinson's. However, only about 10% of Parkinson's cases have been linked to a particular genetic cause (for example, mutations in the *Pink1*, *PARK2*, and *PARK8* genes). Most cases have been classified as idiopathic or sporadic, meaning that the cause is unknown.

- ***Sex:*** Researchers have found that Parkinson's affects approximately 50% more men than women. The reasons for this are not known, however.

- ***Smoking cigarettes/drinking coffee:*** The percentage of cigarette smokers who have Parkinson's is less than the percentage of nonsmokers who have Parkinson's. Based on this data, it might appear that smokers are at less risk of developing Parkinson's than are nonsmokers. Of course, the adverse health consequences of smoking would have to be taken into account before you could conclude that smoking is good for you. But even if the adverse consequences of smoking are disregarded, it cannot be assumed that smoking curtails Parkinson's. It might be the other way around: Parkinson's might curtail smoking. People with Parkinson's may have characteristics that cause them to avoid (or quit) smoking.

The same can be said about coffee. The percentage of coffee drinkers who have Parkinson's is less than the percentage of other people who have Parkinson's. But it does not follow that drinking coffee curtails Parkinson's; people with Parkinson's may have characteristics that cause them to avoid (or quit) drinking coffee. I am not aware of any evidence that coffee or caffeine is a useful treatment for Parkinson's.

- *Stress:* Although some experts theorize that chronic emotional stress triggers Parkinson's disease, others say that stress does not cause or permanently worsen Parkinson's.

• • •

Judy Dodge believes that she developed Parkinson's during her childhood in New Mexico, 50 years or so before her symptoms emerged in Washington, DC, in the late 1990s. Judy's father was a horticulturalist who sprayed insecticides on the fruit trees in his orchard and in the family garden. He did not wear a mask or other protective gear.

When Judy's father finished his work in the orchard and the garden, he made no effort to stop Judy, then five years old or so, from climbing up one of the trees that he had just sprayed. Like her father, Judy did not wear protective gear.

There is no way to know now, some 70 years later, whether Parkinson's seeds were planted then. What we do know is that both father and daughter later developed Parkinson's in their 50s. Judy, now older than her father was in the mid-1940s, believes that both genetic and environmental factors account for her having the same disease her father had. Judy says, "Based on my father's experience and my personal experience, I believe that Parkinson's is caused by a combination of genetic and environmental factors."

Judy's initial symptoms surfaced in 1998. Her symptoms were similar to her father's. Judy's left arm did not swing when she walked, and on at least one occasion, she tripped and fell. Judy's symptoms have slowly advanced since then. She has developed a tremor and has lost her sense of smell. Judy's belief that Parkinson's is caused by a combination of genetic and environmental factors is based solely on her father's experience and her own experience. Judy recognizes, of course, that the experience of two individuals is not enough to establish what causes Parkinson's.

In my own case, I don't know why, when, or where I developed Parkinson's. At times I wonder what I might have done, or have been exposed to, that caused the disease. Was I exposed to something during my first 18 months when my family lived on a farm near the Army base where my father was stationed? Was it a chemical in the chemistry set that I played with as a youth? Was it the soil that the Army contaminated when it disposed of World War I–era weapons near what later became my home in Washington, DC? Or was it just the luck of the draw?

I don't dwell on this. From my perspective, the important question is not what caused me to develop Parkinson's, but what I am going to do about having the disease.

Parkinsonism (Atypical Parkinson's)

Parkinsonism refers to the entire group of diseases that have Parkinson's-like symptoms, such as tremor, muscle rigidity, slowness of movement, and balance problems. Parkinson's disease is the most common form of parkinsonism. Yet it has been estimated that 20% to 25% of the people initially diagnosed with Parkinson's disease by a nonspecialist will eventually be determined to have another form of parkinsonism.

Typically, a patient with Parkinson's disease has Lewy bodies in the brain's neurons. When the patient is given dopamine replacement therapy, the symptoms go away. Parkinsonisms, by contrast, have symptoms in addition to typical Parkinson's disease symptoms, and those symptoms do not respond to dopamine replacement therapy.

The following disorders are among those treated as parkinsonisms, sometimes referred to as atypical Parkinson's:

- *Progressive supranuclear palsy (PSP)* is a progressive brain disorder that causes problems with gait and balance. The signs and symptoms of PSP include an inability to move the eyes properly (particularly, difficulty looking down) and alteration of mood and behavior, such as depression or apathy.

- *Multiple system atrophy (MSA)* is a set of slowly progressive disorders affecting the central and autonomic nervous systems. The signs and symptoms of MSA often include poor coordination, slurred speech, blood pressure regulation problems, swallowing difficulties, male impotence, constipation, and urinary difficulties.

- *Corticobasal degeneration (CBD)* results from atrophy of multiple areas of the brain. The symptoms of CBD include rigidity, dystonia (involuntary muscle contractions), balance difficulties, and problems with coordination.

- *Dementia with Lewy bodies (DLB)* is a disorder associated with the same clumps of protein found in Parkinson's (Lewy bodies), but in widespread areas throughout the brain. The pathology of DLB is the same as that of Parkinson's with dementia. The symptoms of DLB include cognitive problems, hallucinations, bradykinesia (slow movement), muscle rigidity, tremor, and shuffling walk as well as memory loss, poor judgment, and confusion.

Some diseases, including PSP, MSA, and CBD, are referred to as "Parkinson's-plus" syndromes because they have Parkinson's disease symptoms plus other symptoms. Parkinson's-plus syndromes can be very difficult to diagnose, and although some respond to high doses of levodopa, there is otherwise no medication that treats them effectively. Because key symptoms may take a long time to appear or may never appear at all, a movement disorders specialist may need to follow the patient for several years in order to make a definitive diagnosis.

Currently, atypical Parkinson's is diagnosed by observing the patient's symptoms and evaluating the patient's response to dopamine replacement therapy. If the patient's symptoms do not respond to dopamine replacement therapy or respond only briefly, the patient may have a form of atypical Parkinson's.

Diagnostic techniques are evolving. In 2011, for example, the FDA approved the use of DaTscan, an imaging technology that uses small amounts of a radioactive drug to help determine how much dopamine is in a patient's brain. DaTscan cannot by itself diagnose Parkinson's disease or distinguish Parkinson's from diseases like PSP and MSA that can also cause a loss of dopamine in the brain. However, it can be used to help confirm a diagnosis or to rule out certain other diseases with similar symptoms. DaTscan may be helpful if the patient's diagnosis is uncertain or if the patient has not responded well to conventional Parkinson's medication. A patient who is interested in a DaTscan should consult his or her physician.

CHAPTER 4

Movement Symptoms

PARKINSON'S MOVEMENT SYMPTOMS, including tremor, muscle rigidity, slowed movement, smaller movements, and impaired balance, are addressed in this chapter. Parkinson's nonmovement symptoms are addressed in Chapter 5.

As noted earlier, Parkinson's does not affect every patient in the same way. Parkinson's symptoms, their severity, the order in which the symptoms emerge, and the speed with which the symptoms advance vary from individual to individual. Although Parkinson's movement symptoms often emerge first, this is not always so.

Tremor. Tremor—involuntary rhythmic shaking of the hand, foot, or regions around the mouth—is the most common of Parkinson's symptoms. However, many Parkinson's patients (perhaps 20% to 30% of them) do not have tremor, and many people with tremor do not have Parkinson's.

A resting tremor is a typical Parkinson's symptom. A resting tremor in a limb tends to occur when the limb is at rest rather than when the limb is being used. A tremor of the hand when the hand is in use is considered an action tremor and is not typical of Parkinson's.

A Parkinson's tremor starts on one side of the body and migrates to the other side. In my case, tremor was one of the first symptoms I noticed. Although I initially found the tremor annoying and potentially embarrassing, it did not seriously inconvenience me. It occurred irregularly and was limited to my right arm. Today, over ten years after I was diagnosed with Parkinson's, it still occurs irregularly and is still limited to my right arm.

If I am anxious, my tremor occurs more frequently and is more pronounced. On occasion, I find myself caught up in a classic vicious circle. Not only does anxiety provoke the tremor, but the tremor provokes more anxiety. The additional anxiety stems from my concern that the tremor will call unwanted attention to me or my disease and that others will misinterpret the tremor as a sign of uncertainty or a lack of self-confidence.

When I remember to do so, I generally am able to conceal the tremor by putting my right hand in my pocket (if I am standing) or under a table (if I am seated at a table). Today I practice law on a much reduced basis, and I am far less concerned about how others will interpret my tremor than I once was. Most of the people I encounter are already aware of my condition, and I am not reluctant to tell others about it.

The tremor in my right arm sometimes surfaces while I am walking. When that happens, I usually apply one of several techniques to suppress it. One is to make a fist with my right hand. A second is to press the tip of the thumb on my right hand against the tip of my adjacent index finger to form the letter "O." A third is to twist my right arm so that the palm of my right hand faces the direction in which I am walking. A fourth is to relax my neck and shoulders. Although I do not know why these techniques suppress the tremor, they are usually effective, at least temporarily.

Muscle rigidity. Parkinson's patients typically experience muscle rigidity, that is, stiffness or tightness in the arms, legs, neck, or trunk. This can show up in a variety of ways. For example, the voice of a Parkinson's patient can become soft, slurred, and monotonous; the patient may not gesture when speaking; and the patient's dexterity and walking ability may be impaired. Muscle rigidity also results in small, illegible handwriting, known as micrographia.

In some cases, the face of a Parkinson's patient loses its animation, giving the person a "poker face." I will say more about this below in the section on facial masking.

I have had all of these symptoms. Tightness in my hand and arm muscles has impaired my dexterity, and tightness in my leg muscles has impaired my ability to walk fluidly. My facial expressions and speech are affected as well.

Slow movement. Typically, someone with Parkinson's disease moves more slowly than he or she did before developing the disease. For example, the speed of the patient's handwriting may be reduced; when walking, the patient may not swing his or her arms or may shuffle his or her feet; and the patient's eyes may blink less frequently. Some patients are hesitant to begin (or unable to complete) certain movements. Slow movement is often referred to as bradykinesia, a Greek word that literally means slow movement.

Before I developed Parkinson's, I walked briskly. Today, when I walk on city streets, I walk more slowly than the vast majority of pedestrians. I try to walk more briskly, but find it painful to do so. I also speak, dress, eat, unpack the groceries, write, and organize my office more slowly than I did in the past. Rather than resign myself to being constantly late and under stress, I try to allow myself more time to get things done.

Of course, Parkinson's is not necessarily responsible for every symptom that a patient might have. One of the reasons for my slow walking pace has nothing to do with Parkinson's: I have arthritis—osteoarthritis to be specific—in my feet.

Small movement. The size or amplitude of the movements of a Parkinson's patient is typically reduced. For example, the size of the patient's handwriting, the length of the patient's steps, and the magnitude of the patient's gestures may be reduced. This is sometimes referred to as hypometria—movement short of the person's goal.

Impaired balance and postural instability. Balance problems, which often trigger falls, occur later in the course of the disease. A number of Parkinson's symptoms, such as muscle rigidity, slow movement, and postural instability, increase the risk of falling. It also is not unusual for a Parkinson's patient's center of gravity to move, causing the patient to lose balance. Other contributing symptoms include impaired vision, low blood pressure, and fatigue.

Although aging alone increases the risk of falling, Parkinson's patients are subject to twice the risk that applies to similarly situated people who do not have Parkinson's. Because falls can result in serious injuries, they can significantly affect the patient's mobility and quality of life.

Parkinson's patients sometimes fall backward. This often happens because the patient does not lean far enough forward when standing up or climbing stairs.

Balance problems are difficult for doctors to treat. To prevent falling, many patients rely on physical therapy and use a cane or a walker. A wheelchair is a last resort.

I have not had major balance problems, and I have no current need for a cane, walker, or wheelchair. I do occasionally find it difficult to maintain my balance when I get on a city bus that starts moving before I sit down, or when I get up from my seat before the bus comes to a complete stop. I deal with this problem by sitting down as soon as I can (and for as long as I can) and, when I am standing, by using two hands to hold onto the seat in front of me or to grab the straps dangling from the ceiling of the bus.

On a recent bus ride home, I could not find a place to sit. The ride was unusually jerky, as the bus weaved through and around street traffic. By holding onto a strap, I was able to avoid falling, but I clearly had difficulty standing in place. My predicament was sufficiently obvious to attract the attention of at least one other passenger—a woman in her 20s who offered me her seat. I declined the offer, but I probably should not have. It was the first time anyone had offered me a seat on a bus in Washington, and I was completely unprepared for her unexpected courtesy.

When I climb up stairs, I sometimes feel that my center of gravity is not as far forward as it should be, and I now try to shift it forward. So far this technique has worked, and I have not fallen.

• • •

Since he was diagnosed with Parkinson's in 1993, Dan Lewis has fallen often. Dan is a husky fellow, and when he falls, he falls hard. He tries to avoid falls by using a walker. He wears knee pads to protect his knees when he does fall.

For many years, Dan and I participated in a weekly group session at a voice therapist's office. After one session, I left Dan standing on the sidewalk outside the office building, waiting for his wife to pick him up. I headed to the Metro on foot. Since Dan was using his walker, I assumed that he was not in any jeopardy. I had not gone more than ten yards when I heard someone (not Dan) behind me shouting, "Help! Call 911!" I turned around to see Dan sprawled on the sidewalk and a passerby running to his aid. I immediately ran back and helped him up. Fortunately, Dan was not injured, and I explained to the passerby that a 911 call was not necessary. I have not left Dan standing by himself since.

Dan Lewis: "I tend to fall, for no obvious reason, while standing—such as standing at a support group meeting or standing while waiting for a ride or a taxi. I am aware that I am falling, but I can't say why, and I can't stop the fall. I regularly use a walker. A walker helps me to reduce the number of falls, but even a walker does not always prevent me from falling."

Difficulty walking. When someone without Parkinson's walks, he or she normally takes a step by picking up one foot (the lead foot), with toes up, and then planting the heel of the lead foot in front. The step is completed by pushing off with the ball and toes of the other foot, and the walk continues by alternating this process from one foot to the other.

The normal length of a walker's stride is 40% of the walker's height. When I walk now, my stride is shorter than it once was, and I often shuffle my feet rather than lift them up. When I walk with a shuffling gait, I do not strike the ground with the heel of my lead foot. Rather, I tend to shorten my stride and to slide my feet, one foot after the other.

Often one of the first signs of Parkinson's is a decrease in the natural swing of one of the patient's arms when walking. As the disease progresses, both arms may become implicated. In addition, the patient may have difficulty taking large steps and may develop a shuffling gait.

When I was originally diagnosed with Parkinson's in 2004, I did not swing my arms when I walked. I cannot say whether that was due to muscle rigidity or some other cause. In any event, my arm swing has returned, probably due to my physical therapy regime. I walk for about an hour at least four days a week and make a conscious effort to swing my arms as I walk.

I try to concentrate on my form as I walk. I try to lengthen my stride and pick up my feet and swing my arms. This is not a cure, but it helps. In effect, I am continually relearning to walk. It is a struggle worth the effort. My walking form has improved.

On occasion, I find it difficult to swing my arms in the conventional manner (back and forth in the direction I am walking). When this happens, I swing my arms from side to side (as a speed skater might) and then gradually, after 15 seconds or so, shift the direction back to the standard one. This seems to do the job.

Freezing. "Freezing is a bitch." When Phyllis Richman says this, she is not talking about cold winter weather. She is referring to the times when she cannot walk or continue walking, as though her feet were glued to the floor.

Freezing is uncommon early in the course of the disease, but fairly common later on. It is estimated that 30% to 60% of Parkinson's patients have freezing episodes at some point. In general, Phyllis walks with fluidity. However, she often freezes when she is about to take her first step, when she walks through a doorway, or when she encounters a barrier, such as the furniture in her living room.

Freezing episodes typically last a few seconds or a few minutes. Patients are often able to break a freeze by (1) imagining a line on the floor and trying to step over it; (2) trying to step on a specific tile or mark on the floor; (3) rocking from side to side in order to get started; or (4) using a cane or a walker equipped with a laser pointer that projects a line to step over.

The first two techniques—trying to step over an imaginary line and trying to step on a specific mark on the floor—are similar to techniques I use to improve my walking form. When I walk, I try to take big steps by stretching my legs to reach imaginary or actual lines on the sidewalk.

Impaired dexterity. My dexterity has deteriorated significantly. I can no longer write, type, eat, or button my shirts with as little thought or with as much ease as I could pre-Parkinson's. I have looked for ways to work around these problems. Finding these work-arounds does not require a degree in rocket science, but it does require advance thought.

My handwriting has never been good, but it is now so bad that I frequently cannot decipher what I have written immediately after I have written it. I now type rather than write. Unfortunately, my typing, once passable, has become erratic and inefficient. I find that, unless I look at the keyboard, I am unable to strike the correct keys consistently. As a result, the hunt-and-peck system—looking at the keys as I type—is now often more efficient for me than touch-typing.

Voice recognition software provides an alternative that is far more efficient for me than the hunt-and-peck system. The software allows me to dictate letters, memos, and even draft sections of this book directly to my computer. When I first tried to use the software about ten years ago, it did not always recognize my voice. However, the software has improved significantly since then. As long as my voice is clear, strong, and consistent, the software efficiently converts my thoughts into written words.

Because buttoning my shirt and putting on cufflinks now consume more time than I would like, I allow myself more time to dress than I did pre-Parkinson's. I try to wear shirts that are relatively easy to button, and when I must wear a shirt that requires cufflinks, I try to use cufflinks that are relatively easy to manipulate. As often as possible, too, I wear turtlenecks or other shirts that require no fastening at all.

Another technique is to replace shirt buttons with Velcro. Although I have not used this technique myself, Velcro appears to make it much easier to fasten and unfasten a shirt's cuffs and collars.

My difficulties with writing, typing, and dressing do cause me some inconvenience and frustration. However, because I write, type, and dress in private, these difficulties do not embarrass me. By contrast, I am embarrassed when, in a public setting, I have trouble removing the correct amount of cash from my wallet or manipulating the keys on a key ring. I try to reduce or avoid such embarrassments by using credit cards instead of cash, regularly organizing the cash in my wallet, removing cash from my wallet before I need it, and getting my keys ready in advance.

Facial masking. Consciously or unconsciously, people use facial expressions to communicate feelings and thoughts, such as empathy, approval, agreement, disagreement, or hostility. However, muscle rigidity and slow movement—two symptoms of Parkinson's—cause the faces of many Parkinson's patients to become masked. For example, I often present what some call a "poker face," so that my face offers no clue as to what I am thinking or feeling.

A patient's poker face may mislead people who do not know the patient well and even those who do. They may mistakenly suppose that the patient is unempathetic, bored, unhappy, unfriendly, or downright hostile.

This can happen without the patient's knowledge. It happened to me. A year or two before I was diagnosed with Parkinson's, Joanne and I had dinner with my cousin Sara and her husband at a Washington, DC, restaurant. Sara and I grew up a few blocks from each other in New Jersey, but she and her husband now live in Florida, so this was a family reunion of sorts.

I might not remember the dinner but for Sara's telephone call to Joanne the following morning. Sara told Joanne that I had seemed unhappy during our dinner. Joanne assured her (accurately) that I was not unhappy at all.

Yet Sara's observation upset Joanne. At that time Joanne and I had been married for only two or three years, and we still regarded ourselves as newlyweds. Although we both believed that each of us was very happy, Sara had known me for 60 years, and Joanne was concerned that my demeanor at dinner might have revealed that I was not as happy as I claimed.

Joanne and I discussed Sara's observation and ultimately dismissed it on the ground that I had been distracted during dinner by an unrelated, client-related matter. I did not give the episode further thought until I started to write this book, when it occurred to me that Sara probably *had* detected something: the facial masking that is often a symptom of Parkinson's. As this episode reveals, facial masking can mislead even those who know the patient very well.

The most effective technique for addressing facial masking is also the most obvious one: to remember to smile when it is appropriate to do so. I can smile; I just don't smile without making an effort to smile. The problem with this technique is that it works only if I remember to use it, and I don't always remember to do so.

In some contexts (playing poker or negotiating with a salesman, for example), a masked face can be an advantage. The Parkinson's masked face, however, is worn in *all* contexts—regardless of whether concealing the patient's thinking is advantageous or disadvantageous.

Scott Kragie: "Clients and colleagues observed that I had maintained a poker face in the course of negotiations. These observations were intended as compliments. My poker face kept my adversaries guessing what my position really was. I did not make anything out of the observations: in the context in which I was then operating, being enigmatic was a plus."

Swallowing difficulties. Although this does not tend to occur early in the course of the disease, many Parkinson's patients have swallowing difficulties caused by impairment of their throat muscles. Swallowing requires considerable muscle coordination involving the tongue and jaw muscles, the muscles in the back of the mouth, and the muscles of the esophagus, and slow or rigid muscles can interfere with swallowing. Because food or liquid can get into the lungs, swallowing difficulties can lead to aspiration pneumonia, a frequent cause of death for patients with Parkinson's. (In fact, though, most Parkinson's patients die from causes unrelated to Parkinson's, such as heart disease.)

To head off these problems, I try to remember to take small bites of food and to chew each portion well before moving on to the next bite. This technique is effective when I remember to use it. I have also consulted with a swallowing therapist regarding my intake of liquids. She recommended that I keep my chin down when I swallow. When I remember to do this, it prevents me from coughing or choking.

Like many Parkinson's patients, I also swallow my saliva less frequently than I should, causing drooling. Drooling is not only unsightly and embarrassing; it can also lead to aspiration of saliva—swallowing saliva into the lungs—which can result in pneumonia.

My neurologist has prescribed atropine to alleviate my drooling problem. This medication comes in the form of eye drops, but I use it orally. If I apply a drop of atropine under my tongue three or four times a day, my drooling subsides. Although I find it annoying to be taking yet another medication, it is less annoying than the consequences of *not* taking the medication.

Speaking difficulties. The majority of Parkinson's patients have speech and voice disorders at some time in the course of their disease. The most common problems include soft, hesitant, or slurred speech, poor articulation of words, and running words together. The exact cause of these speech symptoms is not clearly understood.

In my case, my voice became markedly softer three or four years following my diagnosis. I was completely unaware of the change. When Joanne observed that I was not speaking as loudly as I should have and that she was having difficulty hearing me, I thought it was Joanne's hearing—not my speaking—that was impaired.

I should have known better. I had noticed that on occasion my speech was slurred. For reasons I could not explain, I occasionally had trouble articulating words as crisply as I had in the past. I didn't see the connection between the slurring of my speech and the volume of my speech. I was unaware of (or unwilling to recognize) the connection between Parkinson's and the muscle coordination that speech requires.

When my neurologist recommended that I consult a speech therapist, I could not continue to deny what Joanne (and my sons) insisted was obvious: my voice needed help. I consulted a speech therapist, and my voice improved. The value of speech therapy for Parkinson's patients is addressed in Chapter 7.

CHAPTER 5

Nonmovement Symptoms

EXPERTS ESTIMATE that, during the course of the disease, from 70% to 85% of Parkinson's patients suffer from depression, anxiety, hallucinations, delusions, or behavioral disorders. Parkinson's patients cannot choose their symptoms, but these nonmovement symptoms are the ones I most want to avoid. I imagine most other Parkinson's patients feel the same way. Because understanding these symptoms can help, I discuss them in some detail in this chapter.

Psychiatric Symptoms

Depression. Depression is not just a matter of feeling sad. Everyone feels sad from time to time. Sadness is temporary. Depression, by contrast, is persistent. The symptoms of depression include persistent sadness; lack of energy; lack of motivation; feelings of hopelessness, guilt, worthlessness, or helplessness; loss of interest in activities or hobbies; difficulty concentrating; difficulty falling asleep or staying asleep; contemplation of death or suicide; and ongoing aches and pains that do not respond to treatment.

It is estimated that 40% to 50% of Parkinson's patients experience depression during the course of the disease. About half of these patients (20% to 25% of all Parkinson's patients) suffer from major depression; the remainder suffer from a mild form of depression called dysthymia. It is not clear why the percentage is so high. Depression could be the patient's reaction to learning that he or she has a chronic illness, the patient's reaction to Parkinson's-related changes in the brain's chemistry, or both. Fortunately, I have not yet experienced any of the symptoms of depression.

On occasion, depression is the first symptom of Parkinson's, occurring even before movement symptoms appear. In these cases, depression may be due, entirely or partly, to Parkinson's-related changes in the brain's chemistry. As I explained in Chapter 3, Parkinson's causes changes in areas of the brain that produce dopamine, serotonin, and norepinephrine—which regulate mood, energy, motivation, appetite, and sleep.

Both Parkinson's and depression can make the symptoms of the other illness worse. Some experts say that patients who suffer from both illnesses tend to have symptoms that are more severe than those experienced by patients who suffer from only Parkinson's or only depression.

• • •

After Shelly London retired from the practice of law at age 63 in December 2001, he was no longer himself. As Shelly's wife, Marge, put it, he was "no longer the man [he] used to be." Shelly's personality changed gradually. By 2011 he was disengaged, lacking in motivation, and sleeping a lot. Marge thought Shelly was depressed and urged him to see a psychiatrist. Shelly knew something was wrong. He followed Marge's advice and consulted a psychiatrist.

Shelly and the psychiatrist met each Friday morning for two years. The psychiatrist did not mention the possibility that Parkinson's disease was the source of Shelly's problems. Shelly didn't have a tremor or slurred speech—two of Parkinson's more well-known symptoms—but Shelly believes there were signs of Parkinson's that the psychiatrist should have picked up on. For one thing, when Shelly walked, he shuffled his feet. For another, Shelly often had difficulty sitting down and getting up from a chair. Shelly also fell asleep in the adult education classes he was taking; he had never fallen sleep in similar circumstances before. There also were a growing number of very embarrassing episodes of incontinence. In addition, Shelly would get up as many as eight or nine times a night to urinate. Shelly also suffered from erectile dysfunction. As Shelly puts it, his "sexual apparatus wasn't working." This very much vexed him.

After almost two years of unproductive sessions with the psychiatrist, Shelly had two fainting spells. After the second, Shelly found his way to a cardiologist's office. There a young cardiologist immediately suspected Parkinson's and urged him to see a neurologist. Shelly was able to schedule an appointment with a neurologist that very day. The neurologist administered a series of tests and promptly concluded that Shelly had parkinsonism.

Shelly wept. Shelly's tears were tears of joy. At last he had a diagnosis.

An anonymous patient: "Depression was an issue for me early on. I was able to fend it off, however, by working out and by staying busy."

Cassandra Peters: "I suffered from severe depression. When I would come home from work, I would lie down on the couch and wouldn't express an interest in anyone or anything.

"It was a very dark period. I was absolutely bereft. I didn't want to see anyone. I didn't want to go anywhere. I didn't want to do anything."

An anonymous patient: "There is now a flatness in my life, no joy, and a decline in religious interest/belief."

An anonymous patient: "I have very low energy, I sleep excessively, and I get tired very easily."

Anxiety. Anxiety encompasses feelings that range from the feeling that something will go wrong (a mild form of anxiety) to a phobia or a panic attack (an acute form of anxiety) that causes the patient to have a rapid heartbeat, to tremble, and to perspire.

Parkinson's patients often find that they are anxious, nervous, or agitated in situations that would not have bothered them before they were diagnosed.

Anxiety is almost as prevalent as depression among Parkinson's patients. It is estimated that 25% to 40% of Parkinson's patients have, at some point during the course of the disease, significant anxiety disorders, such as phobias about going out in public or being in crowded places. Some patients experience anxiety as a result of their Parkinson's symptoms. These patients may be concerned about how others will react to their tremors, their speaking, walking, or thinking difficulties, or their drooling.

Cassandra Peters: "I suffered from severe anxiety. I was afraid to go out in public. I was afraid to drive. It was completely out of character for me."

An anonymous patient: "I am easily flustered when I am challenged . . . for example, when I am questioned while checking in for a flight at an airport."

Apathy. Many Parkinson's patients have feelings of apathy: lack of interest, low motivation, and indifference. Activities that interested such patients before they developed Parkinson's—their careers, their hobbies, and socializing with their friends, for example—no longer interest them. Getting out of bed (or off the couch) to engage in activity requires them to exert considerable effort. Some patients refrain from engaging in conversation and become withdrawn and socially isolated.

Apathetic patients often appear to others as lazy or uncaring. Some Parkinson's patients do not complain about feelings of apathy because, by definition, they do not care. Often it is the patient's spouse who initially observes that the patient shows no interest in activities or subjects that previously interested the patient quite a lot.

Apathy differs in some respects from depression. People with apathy lose initiative and motivation; they become less active and more passive. They still enjoy engaging in the activities that they enjoyed before Parkinson's came along, but they lack the motivation to initiate those activities.

Fatigue and shortness of breath. "Fatigue" refers to a lack of energy or a sense of tiredness out of proportion to the energy expended. It is not the same as sleepiness, apathy, or depression. It is possible to have fatigue but not depression. However, it is also possible to have both fatigue and depression, and fatigue is thought by some to make depression worse (and vice versa).

About 50% of Parkinson's patients are reported to experience fatigue, often but not always in the early stages of the illness. There are a number of reasons why a Parkinson's patient might feel fatigue. For example, Parkinson's can cause low blood pressure or the loss of deep sleep, each of which could cause a sense of fatigue. A patient also might be fatigued as a result of being over-medicated or under-medicated.

In addition, Parkinson's patients occasionally experience shortness of breath, known as dyspnea. When it is a symptom of Parkinson's, dyspnea responds to medications like levodopa, described in Chapter 7. As with fatigue, however, shortness of breath may have another cause, such as lung conditions or heart failure. A patient who is short of breath should seek medical attention immediately.

Chris Whitmer (a stay-at-home-dad whose wife works):"I lack energy. I can't ski like I used to. I can't throw a football with my son like I used to. I can't play soccer with my daughter like I used to. I nap twice a day, but when my wife comes home from work, I am so tired she has to help with the kids."

An anonymous patient: "I often fall asleep when reading. This is part of my general malaise."

An anonymous patient: "I feel fatigue after any kind of exercise, wholly disproportionate to any effort I put forth while exercising. In addition, within minutes after taking Parkinson's medication, I can fall into a deep sleep for from 1 to 2½ hours."

An anonymous patient: "I am generally very active, but I have very little energy and spend more time sitting around and watching TV."

Hallucinations, illusions, and delusions. Hallucinations involve seeing things that are not really there. Parkinson's-related hallucinations may be fleeting or last for hours. Usually they are strictly visual. The patient might see spots, dots, lines, or other small shapes, or people, animals, or bugs. Hallucinations are not necessarily reflective of dementia, and if they develop, this does not necessarily imply that the patient is becoming demented.

Illusions are similar to hallucinations except that the patient sees things that are actually there, but misinterprets them. Illusions tend to be less troublesome than hallucinations.

Delusions are ideas that have no factual basis or false beliefs that an individual adheres to despite evidence to the contrary. In Parkinson's, delusions often involve false beliefs about the patient's spouse, such as a conviction of the spouse's infidelity.

It is estimated that 40% to 50% of Parkinson's patients experience hallucinations, illusions, and/or delusions at some point during their illness. Often the symptom is a side effect of Parkinson's medication rather than an effect of the disease itself. In such cases, the hallucinations, illusions, or delusions can be stopped by eliminating one or more of the drugs that the patient is taking. In addition, if the patient is susceptible, hallucinations, illusions, or delusions can be triggered by any system illness such as an infection.

• • •

For five years, Sarah Boyer took only Mirapex as a Parkinson's medication. Mirapex (a brand name of pramipexole) has side effects, however, and Sarah had first-hand exposure to several of them: hallucinations, vivid nightmares, and screaming in her sleep. Sarah recalls that she saw squirrels walking around her living room.

So loud and emphatic were Sarah's screaming episodes that when she and her husband, John, stayed overnight in a hotel, the occupants of the neighboring rooms complained to the hotel management that they had been kept awake by the noisy argument in the Boyers' room. Sarah's hallucinations, vivid nightmares, and sleep talking eventually went away. "I guess I just got used to [Mirapex]," Sarah says.

•   •   •

Sandra Ridinger has illusions from time to time. Gazing out of her front window recently, she saw a cow (an actual cow) that looked to her like a bear. She realized at the time that this was an illusion, but that was of very little comfort to her since, she says, it didn't alter the fact that the cow still looked like a bear. Recently, Sandra also saw a fence post that looked to her like a man and a boy. Sandra says that so far, at least, the illusions are only an annoyance. They are worrisome to her principally because she fears they might evolve into dementia.

Impulse control disorders. Parkinson's patients occasionally develop impulse control problems, such as compulsive gambling, compulsive shopping, compulsive eating, and hypersexuality. These problems may be provoked by Parkinson's medications, rather than by the disease itself. In most cases, the problems can be treated effectively with medication adjustments.

•   •   •

Learie Phillip initially relied solely on two medications, Sinemet and Mirapex, for treatment. However, Learie's neurologist neglected to warn him that one of the potential side effects of Mirapex was compulsive behavior, such as gambling.

Prior to that time, Learie's gambling activity had been limited to occasional purchases of lottery tickets and the like. However, after he began taking Mirapex, Learie's interest in gambling became pronounced and obsessive. For more than two years, he regularly traveled to casinos in West Virginia and New Jersey to play slot machines. Sometimes he won, and sometimes he lost, but mostly he lost. Learie's gambling losses mounted. Learie was so embarrassed about the losses that initially he did not tell his wife, Cecile.

At last, Learie told both his neurologist and Cecile about the gambling. The neurologist explained that this was probably a side effect of the Mirapex, and he adjusted Learie's medication. Learie's gambling activity stopped immediately, but he is still angry at the neurologist for failing to warn him.

An anonymous patient: "My impulse control problems include masturbation and compulsive eating."

An anonymous patient: "Since going on Mirapex, I've been on the internet more than usual."

Sleep disorders. Many Parkinson's patients encounter serious sleep problems, including an inability to fall asleep, difficulty staying asleep, the loss of deep sleep, uncomfortable sensations in the legs (often referred to as "restless leg syndrome"), nightmares, acting out of dreams, falling out of bed, sleep apnea (a period of time with little or no breathing), and daytime sleepiness. Some of these problems are caused by Parkinson's itself; some are caused by the medicines that Parkinson's patients take; and some are caused by both the disease and the medications.

Rapid eye movement sleep behavior disorder—the acting out of dreams during sleep—is very common among Parkinson's patients. People who develop this disorder in their early 40s are likely to develop Parkinson's. However, not all persons with rapid eye movement behavior disorder develop Parkinson's.

In some cases, depression—common among Parkinson's patients—may interfere with sound sleep or prevent the person from sleeping at all. Anxiety or depression may also cause a delay in falling asleep or early morning awakening. A patient who believes that anxiety or depression is causing a sleep problem may wish to consult a physician to determine whether an antianxiety or antidepression medication would help.

Excessive daytime sleepiness can be the result of poor sleep at night or a side effect of Parkinson's medications. If medications are the source of the problem, adjusting the medications may be helpful, or another medication may help to combat the sleepiness.

The patient might address insomnia and other nighttime sleep disorders by observing regular and sensible bedtime and wake-up times, by following daily mental and physical exercise routines, by eliminating caffeine after dinner or even in the afternoon, by eliminating alcohol within a few hours before bedtime, and by avoiding daytime naps.

Some patients find that an extra dose of Parkinson's medication or a sleeping medication can help to alleviate sleep disturbances. In other cases, sleep disturbances may be caused by medical conditions unrelated to Parkinson's. For example, a disruption in breathing can also interfere with sleep, and it can be treated separately from Parkinson's. A patient who has these symptoms should discuss them with a physician.

In my own case, I do not have difficulty falling asleep. Staying asleep is another matter. During the period before my DBS surgery, I often arose after only three or four hours of sleep and found that I could not go back to sleep. Rather than awaken my wife, I would leave our bedroom and go elsewhere in the house to read or write until I could fall asleep or until it was time for me to go to the office.

I discussed the problem with my neurologist. He hypothesized (correctly, it turned out) that my sleeping problem stemmed from my medications rather than from Parkinson's itself. After we modestly adjusted the medications I was taking, I found that staying asleep through the night was no longer a problem.

Other sleep-related problems have not been so easily resolved. Rapid eye movement sleep behavior disorder can cause a patient to act out his or her dreams, yell, scream, kick, punch while sleeping, or fall out of bed. In my case, unfortunately, these problems—nightmares and the acting out of dreams—have had a direct effect on my wife. Joanne reported that my sleep talking was loud, emphatic, and filled with profanity, and that I was flailing away—sometimes at her! Joanne was not exaggerating: I awakened in the midst of two of these episodes to find that I was punching her. Luckily, this has not happened often.

On several occasions, I have also fallen out of bed while sleeping, the most recent falls occurring in 2013 and early 2016. In the 2016 episode, I injured myself by banging my head against a small chest next to our bed. The injury was just a minor wound, but there is no assurance that I will be so lucky the next time. I plan to discuss this with my neurologist. The principal options appear to include changing the furniture in our bedroom and changing my medication. Experts say it is not clear how often Parkinson's patients fall out of bed because patients often don't report it and doctors don't routinely ask about it.

My internist has recommended that I consult a sleep specialist to assess whether I suffer from obstructive sleep apnea, which is often associated with snoring and excessive daytime sleepiness. The sleep specialist performs an overnight "sleep study" to determine whether the patient has sleep apnea. The condition is typically treated by subjecting the patient to continuous positive airway pressure (CPAP), administered by a mask that fits over the patient's mouth and nose. A tube connects the mask to a machine that creates enough pressure to keep the airway open. I do not think that I have sleep apnea, and I have not yet acted on my internist's recommendation.

Dan Lewis: "I have very serious sleep problems if I don't take my medications—clonazepam and trazodone. I get up at 2 a.m. and can't go back to sleep."

Pete Riehm: "The CPAP provided Maggie with immediate relief [from my snoring]."

Social isolation. Many Parkinson's patients refrain from socializing. Socialization often requires travel, and because Parkinson's can restrict a patient's mobility, the disease can make it difficult to travel.

In addition, many Parkinson's patients are reluctant to socialize because voice problems make it difficult for them to communicate. Other patients are embarrassed by their physical
symptoms, such as tremors and drooling. Still others are handi-
capped by cognitive deficiencies, apathy, anxiety, fatigue, or depression. Social isolation masks rather than addresses these
problems and, by so doing, expands the adverse consequences of
the disease.

Bonnie Kramer: "Michael [Michael Rosenbush, Bonnie's late
husband] hated Washington. He hated the self-importance
and the puffery that he saw in so many Washington people. By contrast, in the support group he found a community with which he felt comfortable. Members of the group
exercised together, laughed together, and commiserated
together."

Bert King: "If you have Parkinson's, you have to fight the tendency to become isolated. You have to push yourself every
day. You have to make the effort to maintain social contacts.
I am active on the board of the Parkinson's Foundation; I am
active in my synagogue; I am active in my condominium. My
life is as full as I want it to be."

Cognitive Symptoms

As Parkinson's advances, many patients experience a decline in
cognition, the mental abilities involved in retrieving, process-
ing, and using information. Parkinson's can make it difficult for a
patient to remember or to process information or to concentrate,
and it can impair the patient's executive function skills (those
used in planning, initiating, and following through on tasks,
problem-solving, and multitasking).

In some cases the decline in cognition is so subtle that it has
no effect on the patient's daily routine. In other cases, the decline
is pronounced. Many Parkinson's patients worry about possi-

ble cognitive impairment in their future. Whenever my memory fails me (for example, because I can't remember that the capital of South Dakota is Pierre), I wonder whether I am having a cognitive symptom. So far, I have no good reason to think that I am.

Some types of cognitive training may help to mitigate the symptoms of Parkinson's patients. These will be discussed in Chapter 7.

Dementia. Dementia refers to a persistent decline in the patient's cognitive function that impairs the patient's ability to engage in commonplace daily activities so that, for example, the patient is no longer able to balance a checkbook.

Some reports indicate that about 25%, or even 33%, of patients with advanced Parkinson's develop dementia. However, the majority of Parkinson's patients do *not* develop dementia, and when dementia does appear, it is typically late in the course of the disease.

Of course, some people who do not have Parkinson's are demented, and older people in particular are subject to the risk of becoming demented. However, the increased risk of dementia for those who do have Parkinson's is significant, and for me this is probably the single greatest concern about having Parkinson's. I fear that if I become demented, I will become a less capable, less independent person. I have always taken pride in my ability to take care of myself and my family, financially, emotionally, and physically. Because Parkinson's could take that capability away from me, it threatens my sense of who I am.

My neurologist told me that there are degrees of dementia, and that a patient who has only "mild" dementia is far better off than a patient with severe dementia. This information is helpful, though it does not eliminate my concern.

• • •

Although most Parkinson's patients report that their initial symptoms were movement symptoms, several of the patients I interviewed reported that their initial symptoms were cognitive in nature. One anonymous patient (a lawyer) said that, in the year

2000 or thereabouts, he began to have difficulty concentrating—a potentially significant problem for a lawyer. For example, he would be reading a regulation, and by the time he reached the third section, he would forget what the first section provided.

Initially, this patient was able to overcome such obstacles by adopting what he calls "coping mechanisms." In the case of a regulation, he would simply go back and re-read the first section to recall what it provided. It was a time-consuming and arduous process, but he found it tolerable. He also coped, he says, "by taking more copious notes. It got to the point where, if I was going to have a conference call, instead of having a yellow pad with five bullet points on it, I had a detailed outline put together, which was a coping mechanism. I was trying to compensate."

Eventually this patient retired. As his concentration problem became more severe, it was increasingly difficult and time-consuming for him to use coping mechanisms. He was working harder and harder, and his efforts were on the verge of spiraling out of control. He concluded that retirement was the sensible choice.

● ● ●

By contrast, when Pete Riehm was diagnosed with Parkinson's in 2009, his initial symptoms were movement symptoms. In late 2014, however, Pete found that his math and concentration skills were deteriorating. Math had always been his strong suit, and it frustrated Pete that he could no longer balance the family checkbook in his head. He had been proud of his math skills. "It was the essence of me," he says. "I wonder what else is coming along . . . It's frustrating for me, and it's frustrating for [Maggie, his wife]. So I know I'm affecting two people."

Dual task interference. Parkinson's interferes with the performance of individual tasks, such as speaking, swallowing, walking, and talking. In everyday life, however, we do not always perform these tasks separately; we often perform two or more tasks simultaneously. We speak, and we swallow. We walk, and we talk. We multitask.

If Parkinson's makes it difficult to walk, Parkinson's makes it even more difficult to walk and to carry on a conversation at the same time. For example, if a Parkinson's patient talks to a companion while taking a walk, the patient may be more likely to fall.

Dual task interference has been studied by having patients do mental arithmetic while walking. The study showed that the patients' walking deteriorated when they did the mental math.

When walking requires an unusual amount of effort, I often find it difficult to carry on a conversation at the same time. The effort I exert when walking up a hill, for example, seems to interfere with the effort I need to carry on a conversation. The two tasks seem to draw on the same limited pool of energy.

Parkinson's also seems to make it more difficult for me to switch my attention from one task to another. When I am concentrating on one task (for example, when I am completing a Sudoku puzzle), I find interruptions more disturbing than I did before I was diagnosed with Parkinson's.

Similarly, Trisha Clark observes that her partner, Ivan Brown, doesn't respond or react to questions as quickly now as he did before developing Parkinson's. She says that she reminds herself that this is a symptom of the disease, not evidence of inattention.

Dan Lewis: "At times, I have problems with . . . executive function. I can't deal with calendar issues. I am hopeless about that. I am never sure what day it is. I have problems with proper names. Before Parkinson's took over, I could go to court and speak to the judge fluently, in well-organized sentences and paragraphs on the basis of ten words that I had written down on a piece of paper. I haven't completely lost the ability to speak like that, but I need to prepare a lot more now. I used to be able to speak, off the cuff, in perfect sentences and paragraphs. It bothers me that I can no longer do that."

Wilma Hazen: "Chuck [Linderman, her husband] has changed. He used to be a take-charge guy. Now he is more tentative. He puts matters off."

Autonomic Symptoms

Alpha-synuclein—the protein that clumps in the brains of all people with Parkinson's—has been found in several locations outside the brain, including the nerves controlling the intestines. Some researchers have raised the possibility that alpha-synuclein shows up in these nerves first, causing nonmovement symptoms, and later spreads to the brain to cause movement symptoms.

Parkinson's patients often develop problems in the autonomic nervous system—the largely unconscious system that controls our body temperature, pulse rate, blood pressure, bowels, bladder, sweat glands, and sexual function, among other things. The autonomic nervous system monitors the body's internal systems and makes adjustments to meet the body's needs. For example, when the autonomic nervous system senses that the body is too hot, the body sweats.

Constipation. Almost 80% of Parkinson's patients have constipation. Constipation means that bowel movements become difficult, infrequent, or both. Since the normal interval between bowel movements varies from individual to individual, it is not possible to state categorically when the interval is excessive. My internist has told me that I should have at least three or four bowel movements a week. So far, I have met that standard.

The fact that a Parkinson's patient is constipated does not mean that Parkinson's caused the constipation. Some of the medications used to treat Parkinson's, mainly anticholinergic medications, can cause constipation (see Appendix 4). Constipation can also be caused by something else, such as not drinking enough water, a diet that is low in fiber, lack of exercise, travel or another change in daily routine, or other medical problems. Appropriate changes in diet and lifestyle are often the most effective therapies.

Urinary dysfunction. Some patients have problems with bladder frequency—feeling the need to urinate often. Others have problems with bladder urgency—feeling the need to urinate immediately. Both conditions may lead to incontinence.

There are a number of ways to deal with incontinence, including incontinence pads and clothing that is easy to remove in the bathroom. In order to limit the number of nighttime trips to the bathroom, a patient also may find it helpful to limit fluid intake in the evening.

Medication can also help. Shelly London, a patient mentioned earlier in this chapter, reports that as a result of taking Sinemet, he awakens each night to urinate no more than once or twice, far fewer than the eight or nine times he was awakening on occasion beforehand. This, Shelly says, was a "magnificent accomplishment."

Sarah Boyer: "Before being diagnosed with Parkinson's, I had repeated episodes of bladder urgency. I mistakenly assumed that a urinary tract infection was the source of the problem. Not until several years later, when I was diagnosed with Parkinson's and started taking Mirapex, did the episodes subside."

Low blood pressure. For a Parkinson's patient, a low standing blood pressure is usually attributable to a combination of an abnormal autonomic nervous system and the effect of medications. The autonomic nervous system ordinarily stabilizes blood pressure when an individual stands up from a sitting or reclining position. This function can be impaired by Parkinson's. In addition, Parkinson's medications tend to cause orthostatic hypotension, a drop in blood pressure when a person stands up. If a Parkinson's patient has a severe drop in blood pressure when standing up, the patient could black out and fall.

A neurologist told me about male patients who deliberately dehydrated themselves to avoid incontinence. In so doing, the patients made their orthostatic hypotension worse, increasing the risk of a fall and a fractured hip.

One way of dealing with low blood pressure is simply to rise more slowly from a sitting or reclining position. Another is to wear abdominal binders or supportive elastic stockings that reduce the amount of fluid that pools in the legs when sitting or reclining. Medications that treat orthostatic hypotension are also available.

· · ·

Joel Havemann was diagnosed with Parkinson's in 1989 and had DBS surgery in 2004. Joel's symptoms advanced gradually until 2012, when he had a series of falls. Joel fell on approximately eight occasions in that year, "cracking [his] head open" twice. Joel believes that dizziness brought on by low blood pressure accounted for at least two of the falls.

When Joel's neurologist recommended that he use a walker, Joel initially resisted, saying that he "didn't want to be typed." In 2013, however, Joel relented and began using a walker. Even with that aid, however, Joel has difficulty maintaining his balance and falls from time to time.

Sexual dysfunction. Patients of both genders report a loss of desire and an overall dissatisfaction with their sexual life. Male patients report erectile dysfunction and problems with ejaculation, while female patients report loss of lubrication and involuntary urination during sex. It has been estimated that 60% to 80% of Parkinson's patients experience sexual dysfunction at some point during the course of the disease.

A number of Parkinson's symptoms, such as tremor, muscle rigidity, depression, drooling, and a lack of dexterity, can interfere with sexual function. Physical activity and appropriate treatment of depression can help to resolve some sexual problems.

A Parkinson's patient should discuss any sexual problems with his or her primary care physician or neurologist. The doctor may refer the patient to a urologist or a gynecologist for evaluation.

An anonymous patient: "I have low libido and cannot maintain an erection."

An anonymous patient: "I have erectile dysfunction and am unable to climax. There is a disparity between great desire and no performance."

An anonymous patient: "I have a difficult time maintaining an erection. I would like to have a four-hour erection [a wry reference to a warning, in a television commercial for a medication for men with erectile dysfunction, about four-hour erections]."

Skin disorders. Many Parkinson's patients develop skin problems, including oily or flaking skin, dry skin, or excessive (or insufficient) sweating. Melanoma, the most serious form of skin cancer, also appears to develop more frequently among Parkinson's patients than among the general population. For this reason, neurologists recommend that Parkinson's patients consult a dermatologist for regular skin examinations.

Many Parkinson's patients develop seborrheic dermatitis. "Seborrhea" is oiliness of the skin. "Dermatitis" refers to inflammation of the skin. Seborrheic dermatitis is a skin condition marked by oiliness, redness, and scaling of the skin especially on the face, the sides of the nose, eyebrows, eyelids, and over the ears. It may also occur in other areas where there is a high density of oil glands, such as the armpits, under the breasts, the groin, and buttocks.

It is not known why Parkinson's patients tend to develop seborrheic dermatitis. Some theorize that it is triggered by the autonomic nervous system, which regulates certain chemical events in the skin. Others believe that seborrheic dermatitis develops because Parkinson's disease makes grooming more difficult.

Parkinson's patients can also develop extremely dry skin. In addition, many Parkinson's patients have trouble with too much sweating, while others perspire too little. Both excessive and insufficient sweating may be side effects of Parkinson's medications.

Sensory Symptoms

Pain. Many Parkinson's patients experience pain due to muscle rigidity or muscle spasms, abnormal postures, or reduced flexibility or mobility. Pain is often felt in one area at a time: a shoulder, an arm, calves of the legs, or the neck. Cramping in the leg muscles, especially at night, is a frequent complaint. Another common complaint relates to unusual burning, stinging, or stabbing pain. Some patients also feel unusual tingling or burning sensations.

Personally, I have not had much pain that I can attribute to Parkinson's. Occasionally my leg muscles cramp at night, but this does not occur more than three or four times a year. More frequently, perhaps once a day, the muscles in my hands cramp. This has occurred more often in recent years than in the years shortly after I was diagnosed.

In addition, I have had lower back pain for many years, starting long before I was diagnosed with Parkinson's. Although I do not associate this pain with Parkinson's, it is possible that Parkinson's makes the pain more acute.

Pete Riehm: "When I was first diagnosed with Parkinson's, a nurse told me to 'be prepared for random pains, in random locations, for random reasons, for random lengths of time,' and I have found that to be true."

Ivan Brown: "When my medication wears off, I often feel muscular pain that engulfs my entire abdomen area."

Diminished sense of smell. Although most people with a diminished sense of smell do not have Parkinson's, most Parkinson's patients have a diminished sense of smell. The sense of smell may be lost or reduced before the patient has any of Parkinson's movement symptoms. That is exactly what happened to me. I don't know when my sense of smell declined, but I believe that it happened well before I had movement symptoms.

Other patients also recall that they lost their sense of smell long before other Parkinson's symptoms surfaced. Both Bert King and Pete Riehm say that they lost their sense of smell 20 or 30 years before they were diagnosed. Now, with the benefit of hindsight, they believe it might have been the first sign that they would develop Parkinson's.

It is not known why Parkinson's patients are inclined to lose all or part of their sense of smell or why they do so relatively early in the course of the disease. One theory is that Parkinson's is caused by respiratory viruses or inhaled toxins that enter the brain through the nose and that, as a result, the olfactory bulb (the part of the brain involved in the sense of smell) is the first brain structure to exhibit signs of damage.

Because a loss or reduction in the sense of smell affects the sense of taste and diminishes the appreciation of flavor in foods, it may contribute to weight loss. That has not happened to me, however. My appetite is as good as ever.

Impaired vision. The retina—the light-sensitive tissue lining the inner surface of the eye—contains dopamine cells, and when Parkinson's reduces the supply of dopamine, the patient's vision may be affected. In addition, vision is sometimes impaired by a slowdown in the eye muscles, making it difficult for the patient to follow a line of print while reading. Some patients have double vision or blurred vision and changes in depth perception, impairing their ability to read, walk, and maintain balance. Reduced eye blinking may also cause the eyes to become dry and irritated.

Ironically, Parkinson's has, at least indirectly, caused one of my eyes to feel more comfortable. From about age 14 until about age 64, I wore a contact lens in my left eye from morning to night. Putting in a lens each morning required dexterity, however, and my diminished dexterity made it increasingly difficult to put the lens in my eye. As a result, I now wear glasses instead, and my left eye feels more comfortable than it has in years.

Bert King: "This is not the sort of disease for which a doctor can simply prescribe a pill or recommend a course of action, and you're done with it. The patient must become educated and figure out what he needs to do. The patient must assume responsibility for his own care. Three different ophthalmologists told me that my vision problems had nothing to do with Parkinson's. From my reading I was certain they were wrong. Finally, I found a neuro-ophthalmologist who understood the impact of Parkinson's on my vision and who was able to help me."

Loss of Bone Mass

The risk of osteoporosis—the loss of bone mass—can be a major concern to Parkinson's patients. A recent study showed that 51% of female Parkinson's patients have osteoporosis, compared to 25% of women without Parkinson's. Although osteoporosis is often regarded as a "women's disease," the study found that 29% of male Parkinson's patients have osteoporosis, as opposed to 7% of men without Parkinson's. The higher risk of osteoporosis is especially disquieting because Parkinson's patients also have an increased risk of falling. If a patient falls, osteoporosis increases the risk of a fracture.

Osteoporosis is a condition of aging, and Parkinson's patients tend to come from an older segment of the population. In addition, while physical exercise helps to maintain bone strength, Parkinson's patients tend to be sedentary. Furthermore, although milk also helps to maintain bone strength, some Parkinson's patients who are being treated with levodopa reduce their intake of milk (a good source of protein) on the ground that the intake of protein could cause less levodopa to reach the brain. (See Chapter 7.)

Because of these interacting risks, many neurologists recommend that men and women have regular bone health checkups.

CHAPTER 6

Living with Parkinson's

PARKINSON'S CAN DISRUPT the lives of patients and their families. Parkinson's can require families to reallocate responsibilities among family members, to modify housing and employment arrangements, and to make major financial sacrifices. In this chapter I examine both these disruptions and the ways in which patients and their families manage to cope with them.

Family Members' Responsibilities

When asked how he has remained optimistic in trying circumstances, Joel Havemann mentions one word. The word is not "medicine" or "exercise" or "surgery." The word is "family." He refers not only to his wife but also to his children: they have been of "enormous support" to him.

When asked what advice he would give to a newly diagnosed Parkinson's patient, Joel says, with a smile, "Maintain good relations with the members of your family. You might need them some day."

Family frequently plays an underappreciated role in both the patient's diagnosis and the patient's care and treatment. The spouse is often the first to identify the patient's symptoms and to urge the patient to get appropriate medical attention. The spouse also assumes many of the responsibilities for the patient's care and treatment.

Just as each patient's case is different, so it is with each family's response. This is so not only because each family responds to the patient's particular symptoms and circumstances, but also because each family's history influences its response.

My family illustrates the point. I was divorced in 1982. Joanne was widowed in 1992. Joanne and I married in December of 1999, just four and a half years before I was diagnosed with Parkinson's. Each of us brought two sons to our family. My sons, David and Adam Vine, were born in 1974 and 1979, respectively. Joanne's boys, Brian and Todd Levin, were born in 1984 and 1988, respectively.

In 1992 Joanne was only 39 and living in San Diego when her husband, Larry, died at age 43. Larry had been diagnosed with stomach cancer the year before, and Joanne spent the following 11 months taking care of him and watching him die. The experience was wrenching.

Joanne was left alone to raise two young boys. At the end of 1993, she and the boys moved from San Diego to North Potomac, Maryland, a suburb of Washington, DC, to be near her sister, Gayle, who lived in nearby Rockville with her husband and two daughters. There Joanne sought to recover some of the peace, normalcy, and balance that she had lost when Larry died.

In 1995, 18 months after Joanne's arrival in Maryland, however, Gayle died as a result of a particularly aggressive form of breast cancer. The deaths of Larry and Gayle within a period of less than 3½ years left Joanne with scars that made her particularly sensitive to any health problems that I might have.

Joanne was the first to react to my tremor. As soon as she noticed it, she considered it potentially serious and urged me to have my physician examine it. Given Joanne's history, her reaction was hardly surprising.

I initially dismissed Joanne's concerns as exaggerated. As months went by, however, and my tremor surfaced with greater frequency, it became more difficult for me to continue to dismiss Joanne's worry.

When I reported my physician's tentative diagnosis of Parkinson's to her, Joanne kept a stiff upper lip and kept her feelings to herself. However, as she later told me, she was devastated. Even after I was examined by a neurologist who told us that the future course of the disease was unpredictable, Joanne saw history repeating itself and feared the worst: an immediate change in our lives, multiple trips to the hospital, more and more bad news from the doctors, and my early death. Joanne was overwhelmed by the prospect of being widowed a second time before she was 53. While I continued to go to work each day, Joanne, unbeknownst to me, spent each day privately in tears, certain that she was destined to take care of another dying husband. Previously, it had not occurred to her that I might predecease her. My parents were still alive, and Joanne had assumed that, like my parents, I would live to a ripe old age.

Larry's death had pulled the rug out from under Joanne. When I asked Joanne to marry me, she thought I would offer the security that had eluded her in the past. After the Parkinson's diagnosis, she was convinced that her security was illusory.

Joanne now regards my DBS surgery as a turning point—not only in my encounter with Parkinson's but in hers as well. After the surgery, my symptoms stopped advancing, and Joanne gradually began to recognize that the future was not as bleak as she had imagined. Joanne's fear that she would have to take care of a dying husband—a second dying husband—subsided.

Throughout, Joanne has largely concealed her fears and supported my battle against Parkinson's. Recognizing that I do not want her to pamper me, she has gone out of her way to avoid doing so. Joanne knows that I will ask for her help when I want it. For example, I do not want her to zip up my winter jacket or to button my shirt unless I ask for her help. She recognizes that although I do things more slowly now, I want to do them and usually can do them.

Ideally, caring for the patient should not be the partner's full-time job. Many partners already have jobs of their own. Joanne, for example, teaches English as a second language to adults. In addition, partners need time to relax, to pursue other interests, and to sleep. Moreover, many partners have health problems of their own that they need to address. Joanne is no exception. Joanne has Crohn's disease, a chronic inflammatory bowel disorder. Like Parkinson's, Crohn's requires considerable time and attention. For now, that must be Joanne's priority, just as Parkinson's is mine.

In 2007 Joanne published a book, *I'm Still Standing*, a moving account of the central events of her adult life, including our family's encounter with Parkinson's disease. Writing the book was a form of therapy for her and a source of inspiration for her readers. Many of the qualities that she displayed in her book—commitment, honesty, and courage—help to sustain me in my battle against Parkinson's.

In general, Parkinson's progresses slowly and steadily, not suddenly or abruptly. Even though Joanne and I know this, we often find ourselves looking for signs that I have reached a turning point. Every time I slip, every time I drag my feet more than I usually do, every time I struggle to find the right word, Joanne and I wonder whether this is a point at which I begin to lose my battle with Parkinson's. I understand, however, that Parkinson's progresses gradually, not suddenly, and that I can't control Parkinson's. For now I go on, undeterred by what I hope is a temporary setback. I know that my determination helps Joanne too.

As the disease progresses, the patient typically needs more help. Some patients need help not only with driving, grocery shopping, and bill-paying, but also with dressing, eating, and bathing. Helping a patient can be time-consuming, costly, and physically and emotionally draining. Patients sometimes feel guilty about burdening their partners with tasks that, the patients believe, should be the patient's responsibility.

Many partners make major emotional, financial, career, and other sacrifices in order to care for Parkinson's patients. Because partners do not have Parkinson's disease themselves, however, they do not receive expressions of sympathy and support comparable to those that patients receive. It is not surprising that, in some cases, the partner feels frustrated or angry, nor is it surprising that the partner subsequently feels guilty about having these feelings.

Although frustration, anger, and guilt are understandable and natural, they are heavy burdens for a patient or a partner to carry. A number of the patients and partners I interviewed recommended fending off such feelings by sharing them with family, friends, and support group members; by obtaining professional counseling; by allowing or requiring the patient to do more; and by enlisting the help of friends and family.

Patients

Shelly London: "I don't give Marge [my wife] enough credit. Her support has been essential."

Pete Riehm: "If anyone is put-upon by Parkinson's, it is the partner, not the patient. Maggie has her own problems plus mine. She has her own problems because she is a person. She has the problems of Parkinson's because of me."

Glenn Roberts: "I understand that having Parkinson's is like getting hit by lightning. I also understand that I did nothing to make myself vulnerable to this disease. But I still feel responsible for the burdens the disease imposes on Kitty [Glenn's wife]."

Chris Whitmer: "Our kids [ages 11 and 13] have matured sooner as a result of my having Parkinson's. They help out a lot more than they otherwise would. They make their own lunches; they do the dishes; they don't whine; and they don't complain when I ask them to do things."

Partners

Bob Burton: "Regardless of the burdens that Parkinson's requires a caregiver to bear, it is much more difficult for the patient."

Judy Havemann: "I hate doing paper work, I hate finances, and I hate changing light bulbs and trying to fix toilets, but these are minor things compared to what [Joel] had to go through. . . .

"The children have been great. It probably changed their teenage years some. . . . Our younger three kids never [rebelled as teenagers], partly because they knew that Joel was sick and that he couldn't deal with being sick and being their dad and doing all of the things he tried to do with them and their being rebellious teenagers. So they didn't rebel. They were always supportive, and their friends were supportive."

Wilma Hazen: "Driving Chuck to all of his appointments, together with all of the other things I have to do, including my own business, is just exhausting."

Bonnie Kramer: "The key is good communication. If communication between the patient and the partner is good, the patient and the partner can address the issues that Parkinson's raises. That is not to say that it is necessarily easy, but it is possible."

Kitty Roberts: "Frustration and anger are virtually inevitable. My advice is to get counseling . . . good counseling."

Driving

Driving is one of the major family responsibilities often affected by Parkinson's. Because Parkinson's may prevent a patient from driving safely, it threatens the patient's ability to work, to socialize, and to function independently.

In the early stages of the disease, when the patient's symptoms may be mild, neither the symptoms nor the medications may impair the patient's driving. However, both the patient and the partner should carefully monitor the patient's driving.

As the disease progresses, it can compromise the patient's ability to steer, to brake, to concentrate, and to multitask skillfully and promptly. In addition, Parkinson's medications can have side effects, such as sleepiness, dizziness, and confusion, that affect safe driving.

Understandably, many patients are reluctant to restrict their driving. However, they should consider asking their partners and other companions to assess their driving candidly and to speak up if their driving skills show signs of deterioration. Patients should confer with their physicians, with an occupational therapist, or with the local department of motor vehicles, if they or others have concerns about their driving.

A decision to refrain from driving does not necessarily deprive the patient of independence or doom the patient to isolation. There may be acceptable alternatives, such as walking, public transportation, or taxis, or a spouse, family member, friend, or acquaintance who is able and willing to drive the patient.

The cost of alternative modes of transportation is a consideration, of course. But the patient can also benefit from offsetting savings, such as the reduction or elimination of auto insurance, maintenance, fuel, and other costs associated with driving.

Depending on the circumstances, the decision to drive an automobile is not necessarily an all-or-nothing choice. The patient may be able to drive safely during the day but not at night, or on familiar routes in nonpeak hours but not on other routes or at other times.

The Home

Depending on the patient's symptoms, family circumstances, and financial resources, a patient may want to make his or her home more safe and accessible, or possibly move to another home that is easier to navigate.

If this seems overwhelming, I suggest picking the low-hanging fruit first: start with the easy stuff. For example, consider eliminating clutter in the home by moving (or removing altogether) any loose wires, nonessential furniture, and loose area rugs. Also consider installing extra lighting (including night lights) inside and outside the home.

Experts recommend sturdy and stable furniture. A chair should have a relatively straight back, a firm, shallow seat, armrests, and no wheels. By contrast, low, heavily upholstered couches and chairs should be avoided; it can be difficult for a Parkinson's patient to rise from them without help.

In addition, since most household accidents take place in the bathroom, consider installing grab bars on tub and shower walls, putting a rubber bath mat in the shower or tub, and removing any small throw rugs.

If there are stairs inside or outside the home, consider installing a rail on both sides of the stairway. Make sure that both the rails and any rugs or treads are stable. If the patient's bedroom is located on an upper story, consider moving the bedroom to the first floor.

Of course, an alternative is to move to an apartment or a one-story home. That's what Joanne and I did. In 2012 we moved from a three-story home in the suburbs, where our bedroom was located on the second floor, to a one-story downtown apartment. Although we did not believe that a move was necessary, we thought it would be easier to live on one floor than on three. Moreover, an urban setting has advantages for someone with Parkinson's. City living encourages walking and discourages driving. Joanne and I walk to and from doctors' offices, the gym, restaurants, movie theaters, and our friends' homes.

Both moving and the process of disposing of possessions that we had accumulated over the years were time-consuming and exhausting. Joanne and I are convinced that we were fortunate to do this while we were young enough and healthy enough to make moving tolerable. With the benefit of hindsight, we are very glad we moved when we did.

• • •

Instead of moving, Dan Lewis made major renovations to his home. He converted a room in his basement into a gym; he added a ramped entryway to make it easier to enter the house with a walker or wheelchair; and he installed an elevator.

• • •

Judy Dodge was divorced in 1992 and has not remarried. Judy is self-reliant and has learned to cope on her own with the obstacles that Parkinson's presents. Judy is not disabled, and her neurologist anticipates that she will not become disabled.

While Judy lives in Washington, DC, her children now live in Arizona and California. Because it will be difficult for Judy's children to help her if she becomes disabled, Judy has taken precautions. She moved to an independent living facility that gives her the option of moving to an adjacent assisted living facility should the need arise. In taking this step, Judy was influenced by her parents' decision to move to assisted living before they had to. They did their children a "great favor," Judy observes, making it clear that she intends to do a similar favor for her own children in the event she becomes disabled.

Bert King: "You cannot wait for events to dictate what you do. We moved in 2013 from a four-story house to an apartment. We moved before we had to, so we could take our time and move on our own terms. We like the location. It is convenient to local transportation, a grocery store, and our doctors' offices. The move itself was exhausting, however. It took a lot out of me—emotionally as well as physically. We had to dispose of items that we'd collected over the years and that meant a lot to us. We don't have room for them in the apartment."

Scott Kragie: "Apartment living has never appealed to me in the least. But I recognized that the logic was there [to warrant moving from a house with stairs to an apartment on one floor]. I was deteriorating at a rapid enough pace that I was not jumping the gun."

Chuck Linderman: "We moved to a smaller-sized home . . . all on one floor. We have upgraded it to meet the needs of a Parkinson's patient in the future. We added a ramp from the driveway to the front door and equipped the bathroom for someone who may have to be bathed. We were anticipating future needs, not meeting current needs."

Disclosure

Each patient must decide whether, when, and how to disclose his or her condition to supervisors, co-workers, customers, and clients, as well as to family and friends. The ramifications of disclosure are considered in this section.

Employment. Some patients are concerned that if they disclose their condition to their employer, the employer will look for an excuse to terminate them. Although I cannot say that such concerns are groundless, my experience indicates that many employers take an enlightened approach. Enlightened employers have no interest in terminating productive employees or in violating the law.

An employee who is diagnosed with Parkinson's may find it useful to consult a doctor and a lawyer regarding the employee's rights under federal and state disability laws. A disabled employee who does not want to disclose his or her disability to the employer could be confronted by a dilemma. Not disclosing the condition may protect the employee's position, at least for the short term. Yet by failing to disclose, the employee may deceive the employer (and the employer's customers), give the employer grounds for terminating or disciplining the employee, and cause the employee to forfeit his or her rights under the Americans with Disabilities Act (the ADA) and the Family and Medical Leave Act (the FMLA).

ADA. The ADA prohibits an employer with at least 15 employees from discriminating against a qualified individual with a disability. A "qualified individual with a disability" means an individual who, with or without reasonable accommodation, can perform the essential functions of the position that the individual holds or desires. A disability includes any physical or mental impairment that substantially limits one or more "major life activities." Major life activities include performing manual tasks, walking, standing, concentrating, thinking, communicating, and the operation of major bodily functions (including neurological functions). Courts typically recognize that Parkinson's results in impairments that substantially limit one or more of these major life activities.

The ADA also makes it unlawful for a covered employer to refrain from making reasonable accommodations for the known physical or mental limitations of an otherwise qualified individual with a disability, unless the employer can demonstrate that the accommodation would impose an undue hardship on the employer. In order to be protected by this provision, an employee must *request* a reasonable accommodation from the employer. For example, an employee might ask the employer to provide voice recognition software, a more comfortable office chair, modification of the employee's work schedule, a leave of absence, or time off for medical appointments. The employer is expected to engage in an interactive process with the employee to determine a reasonable accommodation. If there is more than one accommodation that is reasonable, the employer is not required to accept the particular accommodation that the employee prefers.

In order to qualify for protection under the ADA, an employee must walk a fine line. The employee must demonstrate that he or she is disabled—suffering from a condition that substantially limits one or more major life activities—but not so disabled as to be unable, with or without reasonable accommodation, to perform the essential functions of the job. Some people with Parkinson's will be able to meet these requirements and will qualify for protection under the ADA, but others will not. Guidance regarding the ADA is available at www.ada.gov.

FMLA. The FMLA requires an employer with at least 50 employees to allow employees up to 12 weeks of unpaid leave in a 12-month period to care for family members or for their own health needs. As under the ADA, if an employee with a disability (or with a disabled family member) wishes to exercise his or her FMLA rights, the employee must disclose the disability by informing the employer of his or her (or the family member's) health needs. Guidance regarding the FMLA is available at www. dol.gov/whd/fmla.

Disclosure to business associates and colleagues. Disclosure to business associates and colleagues also can present challenging issues. Disclosure to them is a personal choice and depends on the circumstances. A patient may be concerned that supervisors, colleagues, customers, or clients will lose confidence in the patient's ability to do his or her job. Moreover, if the disease is well controlled and does not limit what the patient can do, it may not be necessary to reveal the patient's condition to them.

If, however, the patient's symptoms are readily apparent, it seems advisable to let others know about the patient's condition before they start speculating about it—even if the symptoms do not impair job performance. For example, others may wrongly infer from a tremor that the patient is nervous, from a soft voice that the patient has something to hide, or from a poker face that the patient is bored. If the patient's symptoms do impair job performance, disclosure may be required as a matter of responsibility to the employer, customers, or clients. These people will likely notice the decline in the patient's performance in any event, and they may be more likely to give the patient the benefit of the doubt if the problem is disclosed to them in a straightforward way.

In my case, I decided not to hide the information, and promptly informed the chairman of my law firm's management committee and the lawyers with whom I worked most closely. I did not have any cognitive or other difficulties that would impair my ability to practice law. However, I thought that some symptoms, such as my tremor, would be evident, and if I didn't tell my colleagues about my condition, they might draw the wrong conclusions. I have been told that most Parkinson's patients report that their co-workers react better than expected to the news about the patient's disease. In my case, my colleagues were uniformly supportive and empathetic. I had no doubt that they appreciated being informed, and informing them relieved me of what would have been a great burden.

If a patient does tell his or her employer, co-workers, customers, or clients about having Parkinson's, it may also be advantageous to offer to educate them about the disease. Some of them may be just as ignorant about Parkinson's as I was before I was diagnosed and may benefit from—and be grateful for—the patient's offer.

• • •

Joel Havemann did not try to keep his diagnosis a secret. His tremor had been quite visible, and he wanted to explain the reason for it to his colleagues. At the time of the diagnosis, Joel was a senior editor in the Washington bureau of *The Los Angeles Times*. He asked the bureau chief to circulate the news of his diagnosis on the office's internal e-mail system, together with a request not to make a big fuss about it. The news was indeed circulated, and Joel's colleagues respected the request that they make no fuss.

• • •

Similarly, Ivan Brown told his colleagues at the U.S. Department of Labor about his diagnosis. His rationale was practical: his colleagues would have noticed that something was wrong with him in any event.

Fred Moonves: Fred works as a chef at a grocery store. He says that although he has a "hard time getting things done in the time frame I think I should," the store "has been very accommodating."

Chuck Linderman: "I did not disclose my condition to my employer or my closest friends for three years. At that point it was evident that I had an illness of some sort, and there no longer was any point in trying to keep it a secret. My advice is to keep your mouth shut. As soon as the personnel people [at your place of employment] discover that they have a reason for getting rid of you, they will, and if your friends don't know anything about Parkinson's, they really can't help you."

Friends and family. Outside of the employment context, disclosure decisions also must be made on a case-by-case basis. Although it took me a while to get to this point, I am now forthright about my illness. I do not waste time or energy hiding it. I could not conceal my disease indefinitely even if I wanted to do so.

Not long after I was diagnosed, I informed those closest to me that I had Parkinson's. I assured them that it is not contagious and that, with the exception of early onset Parkinson's, there is little evidence that it passes from one generation to the next. My family had concerns, of course, but sharing those concerns as a family was better than my trying to deal with the disease alone. My sons have joined me at Parkinson's seminars, participated with me in Parkinson's fund-raising walks and noncontact boxing drills, driven me to medical appointments, and commented on drafts of this book.

I did not inform my parents about my Parkinson's, however. At the time I was diagnosed, my father was 90 and had a heart condition; my mother was 83 and suffering from Alzheimer's disease. I was concerned that the news would damage my father's health and confuse my mother. These were judgment calls, and I did not make them lightly. I do not regret my decisions, and I rarely revisit them. My father passed away in 2006, two years after I was diagnosed. My mother passed away in 2010.

Bert King: "My father was in his mid-90s when I was diagnosed, so I did not tell him. I don't regret my decision. It would have been too hard on him. I told my mother after my father had passed. She agreed with my decision not to tell my father. My mother lived until 2015, when she was 98."

Sarah Boyer: "We [women] are very different from the men, most of us. The women [in our support group] immediately blabbed to everybody that they had Parkinson's. The men sat on [the information] for years."

Kitty Roberts: "It is difficult to generalize. Every situation is so different. However, I would generally favor disclosure sooner rather than later. Failing to inform family and close friends promptly could hurt and even anger the people you will need to rely on in the future."

Employment

Many recently diagnosed Parkinson's patients must decide whether to stop working. Each patient must make that decision in the light of his or her individual circumstances. As with many other Parkinson's issues, there is no single correct decision.

Among the circumstances to be taken into account are the patient's symptoms and age, the effect of the symptoms on the patient's ability to carry out his or her job responsibilities, and the patient's financial needs, resources, and personal preferences.

Financial considerations are typically very significant, if not decisive. Depending on the patient's age, current earnings, and financial needs and resources, a decision to stop working may subject the patient or his or her family to substantial hardship. Furthermore, some people identify themselves on the basis of their job or profession. For such people, an unexpected withdrawal from the workforce can be very difficult emotionally as well as financially.

• • •

Because Fred Moonves is responsible for preparing breakfast at the grocery store, he arises at 1:30 a.m. each day, in time to exercise before heading off to work. He arrives at the store at about 3:30 a.m., so that breakfast is ready for customers by 6:30. Before Parkinson's took its toll on Fred, he arrived at the store at about 4:30 a.m. Because he now moves much more slowly than he did pre-Parkinson's, he needs an additional hour to prepare breakfast.

Fred Moonves: When asked why he keeps up such a grueling schedule at age 68, Fred replies, "I need the income." "And the health insurance," he adds (although he is eligible for Medicare).

For some, Parkinson's can make the advantages of early retirement (and the disadvantages of continued work) more evident.

However unexpected or unwelcome early retirement might be, it can provide opportunities for a variety of rewarding activities, including civic, charitable, and recreational pursuits. By contrast, if the patient continues to work, he or she might work past the time when those opportunities are available.

In my own case, I am fortunate in many respects. Thrifty by nature, I was able to save enough to make it feasible to reduce my commitment to law practice at age 65. I now practice law on a much-reduced basis. I represent a small number of clients in connection with a few matters; I write articles for law journals; and I provide advice to my colleagues when they ask for it. It is enough to make me feel active and productive, but it is not so demanding as to prevent me from exercising or from engaging in other therapeutic activities.

• • •

Since his retirement, Scott Kragie has been busy and productive. He exercises physically just about every day. Occasionally, he plays computer-based "brain games" to exercise his mind as well. Scott volunteers at Friendship Place, a nonprofit organization that provides housing, medical, and job training services to homeless people in Washington, DC. Scott also volunteers at Gallaudet University, which he describes as "the preeminent university in the world with programs and services specifically dedicated to accommodate deaf and hard of hearing students."

• • •

Cassandra Peters had to stop working as a paralegal in 2004, two years after she was diagnosed. The job was rewarding, but too stressful for Cassandra to handle after developing Parkinson's.

Joel Havemann: "I worked full-time for about twenty years after I was first diagnosed with Parkinson's."

Phyllis Richman: "I retired [as a restaurant critic for *The Washington Post*] within a year after I was diagnosed. I figured I had limited time and limited energy. I didn't want to spend all my time in restaurants with strangers. . . . And [being a restaurant critic is] a physical job; I couldn't use chopsticks as well as I had."

Financial Pressures

As the discussion of employment suggested, Parkinson's can weaken the financial position of patients and their families by requiring either the patient or the patient's partner to stop working or to shift from full-time to part-time employment.

In many cases, however, time is on the family's side. Parkinson's patients often find that they can work for many years after they are diagnosed. Likewise, many patients never require full-time assistance from their partners. Moreover, because Parkinson's tends to strike older people, many patients have voluntarily retired by the time Parkinson's limits their ability to work. A retired patient is more likely to be concerned about the prospect of increased expenses than about reduced earnings.

Health insurance, Medicare, and Medicaid can help patients and their families to bear some of the additional expenses that they incur. The key word in the preceding sentence is "some." Because of premium payment requirements, co-pays, deductibles, and exclusions, patients may still be required to pay for some of their Parkinson's-related medical expenses. In addition, any increase in a patient's *nonmedical* expenses would probably not be covered by health insurance, Medicare, or Medicaid. These programs are discussed in greater detail in the following paragraphs.

Health insurance. Health insurance does not necessarily cover all of an insured person's medical expenses. Insurance covers only the expenses that the policy specifies. The insured is typically subject to cost-sharing provisions, such as premium payment requirements and co-pays, deductibles, and exclusions. Although the Affordable Care Act (the ACA) requires individual and small group insurance coverage to cover ten categories of "Essential Benefits," the ACA does not require large employer-sponsored group health plans to cover any particular benefits other than preventive care. A large employer-sponsored group health plan is prohibited, however, from imposing annual or lifetime dollar limits on any Essential Benefits that the plan elects to cover.

COBRA continuation coverage. The Consolidated Omnibus Budget Reconciliation Act (COBRA) applies to group health plans maintained by private sector employers with at least 20 employees and by state or local employers. COBRA provides that, when an individual loses coverage under an employer-sponsored health plan as a result of certain events such as termination of employment (for a reason other than gross misconduct), the individual must be allowed to continue coverage under the plan (at the individual's own expense) for a limited period of time. Generally, the limited period of time is 18 months, but that period is extended by as many as 11 additional months (for a total maximum of 29 months) if the beneficiary is determined to be disabled by the Social Security Administration (SSA). In order for a beneficiary to qualify for the extended period of COBRA coverage, the SSA must find that he or she was disabled at some time during the first 60 days of COBRA coverage. The extended period of COBRA coverage ends if there is a final determination that the individual is no longer disabled. The plan is permitted to charge beneficiaries a higher premium, up to 150% of the entire cost of coverage, during the 11-month disability extension period.

Medicare Parts A and B. Medicare provides health care benefits to people who are age 65 or older and for certain disabled people under age 65. There are two principal benefits under Medicare: Part A (Hospitalization Insurance) and, for those who purchase it, Part B (Medical Insurance). Only people who have Part A coverage can purchase Part B coverage. Part B provides coverage for medically necessary doctors' services, physical therapy, occupational therapy, and certain other outpatient services. Part B coverage is also subject to numerous exclusions and limitations, an annual deductible, and numerous co-payment requirements.

Medicare Part C. Under Part C (Medicare Advantage), private insurance companies offer an alternative to Parts A and B. A Part C plan provides all Part A and B benefits. In most instances, a Part C plan provides additional benefits and imposes lower co-payment requirements. The size of the monthly premium varies, depending on a variety of factors, including the private insurance company chosen, the insured person's state of residence, and whether a health maintenance organization (HMO) or a preferred provider organization (PPO) provides the coverage.

Medicare Part D. Part D—outpatient prescription drug coverage—plans are available to those enrolled in Parts A and B or in Part C plans that do not offer prescription coverage. A patient on Medicare might either purchase Medicare Part D prescription coverage or switch to a Medicare Advantage plan that covers the cost of prescriptions.

Although Medicare certainly helps with health care costs, beneficiaries must still pay premiums for physician services (under Part B) and prescription drug coverage (under Part D). Medicare also imposes relatively high cost-sharing requirements, does not limit a beneficiary's annual out-of-pocket spending (as some private-sector plans do), and does not cover some services that are often needed by older Parkinson's patients, such as custodial long-term care.

Some Medicare beneficiaries obtain supplemental insurance to help meet their Medicare cost-sharing requirements. However, the premiums for supplemental insurance can be expensive and beyond the reach of the many older Americans.

Medicaid. Medicaid is a federal-state program that supplements Medicare for qualifying low-income beneficiaries. Disabled people also are among those potentially eligible for coverage. Benefits vary from state to state. Most programs help pay for prescription drugs. More information about Medicare and Medicaid is available on the web site of the Centers for Medicare and Medicaid Services at www.cms.gov.

CHAPTER 7

Today's Therapies

THERAPIES CURRENTLY AVAILABLE to Parkinson's patients are described in this chapter. As science and medicine evolve, so will the available therapies. Therapies that may become available in the future are covered in Chapter 8.

Whether a particular measure is appropriate for an individual patient can be determined only on a patient-specific basis. A therapy that the patient's neurologist recommends, based on knowledge of the patient's medical history and current condition, is far more likely to be helpful than something that someone else, possibly in quite different circumstances, considers useful. Accordingly, if a patient's neurologist recommends a therapy that differs from what is described in any book, including this one, the patient should follow the doctor's advice.

I select the therapies that are best for me in a manner consistent with the guidelines set forth in Appendix 5—based on both the best advice I can get and my own educated judgment. I also seek to implement those therapies in a manner consistent with the guidelines: I try to be positive, persistent, and realistic.

Symptomatic Relief

Most neurologists believe that current Parkinson's therapies treat only symptoms, not the underlying disease. They believe that, although therapies might slow the progress of the symptoms, the underlying disease is unaffected and continues to advance. Parkinson's is not unique in this respect. Very few diseases, other than certain infections and cancers, are "cured." Diabetes, hypertension, and heart disease, for example, are treated symptomatically.

Obviously, however, symptomatic relief can be very helpful. Moreover, depending on how long it lasts, symptomatic relief might not differ very much, in terms of the patient's satisfaction, from complete relief from the underlying disease. In my case, for example, Parkinson's symptoms seem to have largely stopped advancing as a result of my DBS surgery in 2008. Whether this means that the disease itself has stopped advancing is, as far as I am concerned, an open question.

Medications

Decisions about when to begin medication, and what medications to begin with, are highly individualized. The decision most appropriate for one patient is not necessarily appropriate for another. Although some patients are reluctant to begin medication right away, most neurologists appear to agree that delaying treatment may reduce the quality of life and possibly increase the risk of falling.

Unfortunately, a patient's missing dopamine cannot be replaced by simply administering additional dopamine as a drug. This is so because dopamine does not cross the "blood-brain barrier," the lining of cells inside blood vessels that regulates the flow of oxygen, glucose, and other substances into the brain.

In 1967, however, the FDA approved the use of levodopa, an amino acid found in many foods. Scientists had found that levodopa could be transported into the brain, where it could be converted to dopamine. Levodopa transformed the treatment of Parkinson's disease. Since 1967, numerous additional drug therapies have been introduced, including dopamine agonists, catechol-O-methyltransferase (COMT) inhibitors, and monoamine oxidase B (MAO-B) inhibitors. These primary types of medication are discussed in the following sections; for details about individual drugs, see Appendix 4.

Levodopa-carbidopa (Sinemet). Levodopa is currently the most effective Parkinson's medication. It passes from the blood stream into the brain, where it is converted into dopamine. It is combined with carbidopa to prevent nausea and to ensure that the conversion does not occur before the levodopa enters the brain. As the disease advances, the benefit from levodopa may decline, and it has a tendency to wax and wane—a phenomenon known as the "on/off effect."

Potential side effects include low blood pressure, nausea, dizziness, and dry mouth. Other potential side effects are hallucinations and dystonia (involuntary muscle contractions). One notable potential side effect is dyskinesia, or random-looking involuntary movements. A patient with levodopa-induced dyskinesia often appears to be incapable of sitting still or standing in one place. Dyskinesia may affect one hand or foot, one side of the body, or the entire body. It may also affect the patient's face. The patient may seem to be grimacing, writhing, or wiggling.

Dyskinesia can lead to improper foot placement and cause instability. In addition, it can impair coordination and cause the patient to drop things. Some patients find dyskinesia to be particularly annoying. In fact, my unhappiness with dyskinesia was one of my reasons for having DBS surgery, and since that surgery, dyskinesia has not bothered me.

Fred Moonves: "There is a fine line between having tremors and having dyskinesias. There are days when I cross the line. I flail around. My arms and legs move. My weight keeps shifting. I have trouble getting words out.

"My neurologist's assistant recommended a course of action when this happens. She said that in order to negate the effect of levodopa, eat as much protein as you can. It helps. It's not always effective, but generally it suppresses the dyskinesias."

Although levodopa does not cure Parkinson's disease, it reduces the severity of the symptoms and dramatically improves the health and longevity of patients. The mortality experience of Parkinson's patients has substantially improved since 1967, the year the FDA approved levodopa for clinical use. In 1967, a Parkinson's patient lived, on average, 5 to 15 years from the date of diagnosis. The corresponding life expectancy today is 15 to 25 years. Although there is disagreement on this point, many experts say that there is now no significant difference between the average life expectancy of a PD patient and the average life expectancy of people of the same age who do not have PD.[1]

Bonnie Kramer: "When Michael [Rosenbush] was diagnosed with Parkinson's [at age 72], his neurologist assured him that he would not die from Parkinson's. He didn't. He died [at age 77] from endocarditis [an infection of the inner lining of the heart]."

Dopamine agonists. These drugs include pramipexole (Mirapex), ropinirole (Requip), and rotigotine (when delivered from a patch, Neupro). Dopamine agonists stimulate the parts of the brain that are influenced by dopamine. In effect, dopamine agonists "trick" the brain into thinking it is receiving the dopamine it needs. They are not as effective as levodopa in treating Parkinson's symptoms. However, they last longer and help to smooth out levodopa's on/off effect. The potential side effects are similar to (but more severe than) those of levodopa and also include hal-

1. See, for instance, Abraham Lieberman and Marcia McCall, *100 Questions & Answers About Parkinson Disease* (Jones & Bartlett, 2003), p. 20; Johns Hopkins Medicine, What Is Parkinson's Disease?, www.hopkinsmedicine.org/neurology_neurosurgery/centers_clinics/movement_disorders/conditions/parkinsons_disease.html; but also see Allison W. Willis et al., "Predictors of Survival in Patients with Parkinson Disease," *Archives of Neurology*, vol. 69 (May 2012), pp. 601–607, available online at http://archneur.jamanetwork.com/article.aspx?articleid=1149703.

lucinations, illusions, sleepiness, and compulsive behavior, such as hypersexuality, gambling, and eating.

COMT inhibitors. Entacapone (Comtan) is the primary medication in this class. It helps to prolong the effectiveness of levodopa by blocking an enzyme that breaks down dopamine. Also available is a triple combination drug (Stalevo) that combines levodopa, carbidopa, and entacapone. Potential side effects of COMT inhibitors include dyskinesias, diarrhea, orange urine, and other enhanced levodopa side effects. For example, entacapone slows the breakdown of dopamine in the patient's brain, and with more dopamine in the brain, the patient's dyskinesias become more pronounced.

Monamine oxidase B (MAO-B) inhibitors. These drugs include selegiline (Eldepryl or Zelapar) and rasagiline (Azilect). They help to prevent the breakdown of dopamine by inhibiting an enzyme that metabolizes dopamine. Potential side effects include headaches and nausea. When combined with levodopa-carbidopa, these medications increase the risk of hallucinations and illusions.

Amantadine. Amantadine provides short-term relief from symptoms of mild, early-stage Parkinson's. It may also be combined with levodopa-carbidopa therapy during later stages of Parkinson's to control dyskinesias. Potential side effects include dry mouth, constipation, urinary retention, drowsiness, hallucinations, illusions, and discoloration of legs.

In most cases, medications can restore the concentration of dopamine in the brain to near normal levels. More dopamine helps to relieve many Parkinson's symptoms, such as stiffness, shaking, slow walking and difficulty in walking, smaller handwriting, and lack of facial expression. Even if no medication halts the advance of the underlying disease, treatment of Parkinson's symptoms is a major accomplishment.

Personally, I approach my medication regimen quite seriously. Whenever my medications are changed, I ask my physician about potential side effects so that I will not be caught by surprise. I check to make sure that the pharmacy has filled my prescriptions correctly. To make sure that I take the medications on a regular schedule, I carry a pill box with me when I leave home.

I also keep on hand a bag containing a week's supply of my medications so that I can take the bag with me if I am hospitalized or otherwise required to leave home in an emergency. The bag contains a memo describing my health condition and medication schedule.

When I travel, I take an ample supply of medications with me and don't let the medications out of my sight. For example, if I am traveling on an airplane, I keep the medications in a carry-on bag rather than in checked baggage.

· · ·

When Sarah Boyer was diagnosed with Parkinson's, she was relieved rather than alarmed. Sarah knew what Parkinson's was and what it wasn't. Sarah had a master's degree in nursing and had taught nursing for over 25 years. Although she had not known precisely what was wrong with her, she knew that most of the other possibilities (such as stroke, tumor, and brain dysfunction) were more worrisome than Parkinson's. Moreover, once Sarah was diagnosed, she knew she could get treatment.

Sarah's neurologist prescribed levodopa to determine whether Sarah had Parkinson's. The levodopa was effective: all of Sarah's symptoms went away, confirming that Sarah had the disease.

Sarah did not want to take levodopa on a long-term basis, however. She did some research and learned that dyskinesias were among levodopa's potential side effects. Sarah's view was that levodopa was not for her, and she asked her neurologist to prescribe something else. He prescribed Mirapex.

Although Sarah's views regarding levodopa are also held by others, their views are controversial. One study suggests that levodopa, compared to dopamine agonists, offers a greater risk of dyskinesias. One of my neurologists, however, says that the study was flawed and that, in his view, it is appropriate for a patient to start with levodopa.

Sarah takes antidepressants too, but she does not believe that her depression is related to her Parkinson's. "Depression runs in my family," Sarah says firmly. "Parkinson's does not."

Trisha Clark: "I see [Ivan] after the medication has worn off. The difference is like night and day."

Chuck Linderman: "I am not sure how efficacious the meds really are. . . . I sometimes wonder what would happen if I flushed all my medicines down the toilet."

Speech Therapy

Parkinson's can compromise the muscles used in speaking. As a result, many Parkinson's patients find that their speech becomes soft, slurred, or garbled. I was one of those patients.

Initially, I was not aware that my speech had become impaired. My family felt otherwise, however, and I consulted a speech therapist. The therapist used the Lee Silverman Voice Treatment (LSVT) method, which concentrates on increasing loudness to improve soft, slurred, or garbled speech.

The focus of the therapy was a series of voice exercises that I performed each day. The exercises were designed to strengthen the muscles I use to speak and to make it natural for me to use them.

I strengthened these muscles in the same way muscles are typically strengthened: by using them. Each day, I read a speech or an article out loud, repeated ten often-used phrases (such as "Good morning, Mrs. Smith" and "Have a good day") six times each, and said "YAH" as long, as low, and as high as I could, six times each—all with an eight (out of ten) level of effort. Like most patients, I initially thought I was shouting when I spoke at an eight level. I eventually learned that this was a misperception and that, in order to be understood, I had to use that level of effort.

When my speech therapist recommended that I see her several times a week, I complained that she was taking over my life. While understandable, my complaint was misdirected. It was *Parkinson's*, not speech therapy, that was threatening to take over my life. The question was what I was going to do about it.

When I completed the LSVT program, the speech therapist played two audio tapes for me: one of my voice when I originally contacted the therapist, and the other of my voice at the end of the program. I was shocked by the profound difference.

If a patient has speech problems but can't, or doesn't want to, use a speech therapist, the patient might (a) focus on speaking louder and more deliberately, (b) take a deep breath before speaking, and (c) practice speaking in a loud voice at least once a day.

Some Parkinson's patients seek to strengthen their lungs and vocal cords by participating in a singing group. Group activity also helps to counteract the isolating effects of Parkinson's and fosters camaraderie and commitment.

Physical Therapy and Exercise

When I was diagnosed with Parkinson's, my neurologist recommended physical therapy. My eldest son, David, also said that he had heard that exercise was important. I didn't say so at the time, but I thought I'd heard all of this before. Exercise, it seemed, was the popular remedy of choice for every health-related problem. In my mind, physical exercise could not possibly remedy a disease of the brain. I recognized that exercise might make me feel better, but I could not fathom how it could help me address Parkinson's in a meaningful way.

I was badly mistaken. Physical exercise may slow down the advance of major Parkinson's symptoms such as tremor, rigidity, slowness of movement, and loss of balance. Exercise can also help with gait disturbances, freezing, and leg cramps.

In fact, recent studies suggest that physical exercise may improve the functioning of the brain by helping the patient's dopamine work more efficiently. These studies also indicate that early incorporation of physical exercise into a patient's treatment program provides the greatest benefit.

Another recent study showed that rats that exercise produce more dopamine in their brains than rats that do not exercise. This raises the possibility that exercise might help the human brain to produce more dopamine. Exercise is also good for the heart and helps the patient to deal with constipation, depression, and anxiety issues more effectively.

Further, scientific studies show that aerobic exercise enhances factors that may have a protective effect on the brain. For example, aerobic exercise may liberate trophic factors—proteins that promote brain cell survival, somewhat like what fertilizer does when applied to a lawn.

More activity and exercise may help to reduce fatigue by increasing strength and stamina. I do feel better after I exercise. I now treat physical exercise as if it were a medication that my doctor has prescribed. I regard a day without exercise as a forgone opportunity.

There is no single type of exercise that has been shown to be particularly beneficial to all Parkinson's patients. Patients are of different ages and have different capabilities, levels of fitness, symptoms, and preferences. Personal preference is important. Patients should select activities that they enjoy. Sustained commitment is necessary, and it is difficult to continue to engage in an activity that one does not enjoy.

I suggest working with a physical therapist to identify appropriate goals and to design a program to meet those goals. Appropriate goals might include increasing or maintaining muscle strength, muscle flexibility, balance, and aerobic fitness.

Periodically, I consult a trainer who is knowledgeable about Parkinson's. He enthusiastically supports my interest in exercise and helps me to fashion an exercise routine well suited to my condition. In addition, periodic sessions with the trainer help to discipline me, just as periodic tests in school encouraged me to do my homework.

The routine that I generally follow is to walk for about an hour four days a week and to go to the gym on the other days. When I walk, I try to focus on swinging my arms and taking big steps. My routine at the gym includes aerobic, strengthening, and stretching activities, and concentrates on three body regions: upper body, lower body, and trunk (core). For example, one exercise requires me to walk backwards, and sideways, on a treadmill. Another requires me to bounce a medicine ball off a rebounder while standing on one leg. Other exercises are more conventional; for example, I pedal a stationary bike and do stretching exercises.

Because Parkinson's patients tend to make smaller motions than other people, I practice making larger, exaggerated motions. I try to take larger and larger strides when I walk. My objective is to have my body make normal movements naturally.

As I become more comfortable with an exercise, I gradually increase the level of difficulty. My objectives are to be challenged and to have fun. Some would say that this formula should be changed to "be challenged *or* have fun." I get the joke, but I try to have it both ways.

Chris Whitmer: "PD wants you to lie down. You have to fight that. . . . You have to go out every day and be active.

"The best tool [for combating Parkinson's] is working out—physical activity in the gym. I feel better when I go to the gym."

An anonymous patient: "My first tremor was when I was 35. I think the reason I wasn't diagnosed until I was 50 was that I was very active. I exercised like crazy. You name it, I did it. Running, swimming, biking, and skiing."

Scott Kragie: "Physical exercise helps with flexibility, gait, and physical competence quite a bit. I used to walk at 4.5 to 5 miles an hour—which is a good pace. Now that I am more symptomatic physically, I am down to 3.5 miles an hour."

Judy Dodge: "Regular physical exercise is a must . . . an absolute must."

Pete Riehm: "Everyone says that walking is the best exercise. [But] it's hard to be enthusiastic about walking after you've fallen and your face has hit the pavement a couple of times."

Some patients have found helpful the nontraditional forms of exercise described in the following paragraphs.

LSVT LOUD and LSVT BIG. LSVT LOUD is a standardized treatment protocol designed to improve the strength and clarity of the patient's voice. It seeks to stimulate the muscles of the patient's voice through loudness training. LSVT BIG is a physical exercise counterpart to LSVT LOUD. LSVT BIG emphasizes increasing the size of limb and body movements to improve movement skills.

Both programs are designed to increase the amplitude of the patient's actions and to help patients recognize that, even if the actions seem exaggerated, they are within normal limits for speech and conduct.

Forced exercise. Forced exercise is a form of aerobic exercise in which the patient's exercise rate is deliberately increased. The beneficial effects of forced exercise were documented by a Parkinson's researcher who captained a tandem bicycle with a patient on a week-long recreational ride across Iowa. Before the tandem ride, the patient trained by herself on a stationary bike at a pedaling rate of approximately 60 revolutions per minute. During the tandem ride, the captain controlled the pedaling rate and averaged 85 RPM. The captain thus "forced" the patient to pedal about 40% faster than she pedaled during training. After two days of tandem riding, the patient reported significant improvement in her symptoms.

Forced exercise is not limited to bicycling. For example, a rower also can participate in forced exercise by rowing in a double shell with another rower.

Noncontact boxing. Some Parkinson's patients have found that noncontact boxing helps to moderate Parkinson's movement symptoms. In noncontact boxing, the boxers do not punch one another; rather, they punch padded gloves or boxing bags and engage in shadow boxing.

"Rock Steady Boxing," a noncontact program for Parkinson's patients, is modeled on the training regime followed by professional boxers. The noncontact boxing exercises help patients to work on endurance, strength, flexibility, balance, rhythm, and speed. If done with a group, boxing exercises also foster camaraderie and socialization.

I have recently tried noncontact boxing with my stepson Todd. Todd puts me through a rigorous boxing workout that promotes strength, speed, stamina, coordination, and balance.

Dance. Some Parkinson's patients find dance to be a useful therapy for balance, gait, and postural instability. Dance rewards not only strength, speed, and stamina, but also form, rhythm, and style. Dance calls for relaxed graceful movement, for multitasking, and for starting, stopping, and restarting. Of course, dance has social as well as physical benefits.

Tai chi. Tai chi involves a series of slow, deliberate movements performed in a focused manner with deep breathing. It is a low-impact form of exercise and puts minimal stress on muscles and joints. Tai chi has been said to reduce stress, to increase energy and stamina, and to improve mood, posture, balance, flexibility, and fluidity of movement. There also is evidence suggesting that tai chi may help to enhance the quality of sleep, improve overall well-being, and reduce the risk of falls. Studies have shown that tai chi can reduce the risk of falls by seniors by up to 45%.

A recent study found tai chi to be particularly effective for balance in people with Parkinson's disease. Tai chi helps to improve balance because it seeks to improve strength, flexibility, range of motion, and reflexes.

Tai chi helps psychologically as well as physically. Experts say that a fear of falling is one of the best predictors of a fall. Tai chi helps to eliminate that fear by making the individual more self-confident on his or her feet.

Reducing the risk of falls obviously reduces the risk of injury from falls. It may also reduce the risk of getting into an automobile accident. The AAA Foundation for Traffic Safety recently found that older people who have fallen have about a 40% greater risk of getting into an automobile accident than those who have not fallen.

Yoga. Yoga involves gentle stretching movements and poses that increase strength, flexibility, and balance. Poses can be done quickly in succession or more slowly. The most popular form of yoga involves a series of poses with attention to breathing, meditation, and proper execution. Different styles of yoga have different levels of difficulty.

Pilates. This physical fitness system is similar to yoga, but emphasizes the body's core. Pilates is designed to improve balance, strength, flexibility, and posture by emphasizing alignment, breathing, core strength, and coordination.

• • •

When a neurologist told Chuck Linderman that he had Parkinson's, Chuck was dumbfounded. He knew nothing about Parkinson's. He had no idea what he was facing. He did not know what to do or think.

After his appointment with the neurologist, Chuck went back to his office. He did not say anything to his colleagues about the neurologist or the diagnosis.

Chuck had a second appointment that day. The second appointment was with Rob, a personal trainer whom Chuck had been seeing each week for over ten years—primarily to lose weight. Unlike Chuck, Rob knew something about Parkinson's: Rob's mother had the disease. Rob also knew Chuck very well, and knew that Chuck would respond to a challenge.

"Chuck," Rob asked, "are you going to fight this thing or are you going to let it take you down?"

"I am going to fight it," Chuck answered. Chuck acknowledges now that when Rob asked him whether he was going to "fight this thing," he did not know what Rob meant.

But Chuck knows now.

"It means lots of work, lots of hard work, lots of work in the gym," Chuck explains, "and it means not giving in to fear, not checking out." Chuck is grateful for Rob's help. "He's been a good partner," Chuck says.

Exercise, especially rowing, has been Chuck's principal weapon in his battle against Parkinson's. Chuck started rowing about ten years before he was diagnosed. He enjoyed the sport, and once he understood that physical exercise was essential in combating Parkinson's, he saw no reason to stop. A latter-day Rocky Balboa, Chuck makes it his business to engage in some form of physical exercise every day. He engages in physical therapy twice a week, and rows (either on the water or on a rowing machine) three times a week. Chuck has won at least one medal at the Bayada Regatta in each of the last five years, and in one year he won three medals. Held each year on the Schuylkill River in Philadelphia, the Bayada Regatta is a USRowing-sanctioned event for disabled rowers and is one of the largest events of its kind in the world.

"My advice to the newly diagnosed," Chuck says, "is to get your rear end exercising."

Exercise has not made Chuck impervious to the effects of Parkinson's. He is a fierce competitor, not Superman. Chuck now uses a rollator (a fancy type of walker) to get around. In 2013 Chuck developed "dropped head syndrome," a relatively rare condition in which the patient loses the ability to hold his or her head up. Chuck's head bends forward so that his chin rests on his chest. He sometimes wears a brace around his neck, but even with the brace on, Chuck's head leans forward.

Chuck is working hard to reverse the effects of dropped head syndrome. He does a series of neck exercises each day at home, and twice a week he sees a physical therapist who helps him focus on strengthening the muscles in his neck. So far, their efforts have produced only modest improvements.

Yet Chuck continues to feel better after exercising. "I know some might disagree with me [about how much exercising benefits him], but I know I feel better," Chuck insists. "No one can take that away from me."

• • •

Sarah Boyer feels much the same way. Sarah exercises several times a week. She works hard in the sessions. Her exercises focus principally on balance, stretching, and walking. Sarah finds these exercises to be very helpful, and she believes they have enabled her to avoid falls. It has been five years since she has fallen.

• • •

Rick Vaughan plays tennis two or three times a week and takes pride in his determination to continue to play. Although Rick acknowledges that the quality of his game has deteriorated some, he modestly accepts his tennis-playing friends' characterization of his performance as "inspirational."

Occupational Therapy

Parkinson's can make it more difficult for the patient to engage in ordinary daily activities, such as bathing, dressing, eating, and writing. An occupational therapist can help the patient to engage in these activities.

This can be done by improving the patient's fine motor skills, for example, by performing exercises such as picking up coins off a table, playing the piano, or manipulating golf balls.

Alternatively, an occupational therapist may recommend using equipment that helps the patient do what others might do without assistance. For example, if a Parkinson's patient finds it difficult to button shirt cuffs, an occupational therapist might suggest using Velcro instead of buttons. If a patient has difficulty typing, an occupational therapist might suggest using voice recognition software.

An occupational therapist also can recommend ways to make the patient's home safer and easier to navigate. For example, the therapist might recommend the installation of bathroom grab bars, shower seats, and night lights, and the removal of loose area rugs and long extension cords.

Shopping for Therapists

It is often difficult for a patient to find a voice, physical, or occupational therapist with the requisite experience, expertise, and personality. Patients generally find it useful to "shop" for a therapist, rather than to use the first one that is recommended. The appropriate selection criteria will depend on the patient's specific needs, but might include experience and success in working with similar Parkinson's patients, expertise, personality, flexibility, availability, and convenience. If experience in working with Parkinson's patients is a key criterion, the patient's support group is likely to be a useful source of recommendations.

Cognitive Training

Some patients adopt coping mechanisms to work around cognitive deficiencies. For example, some patients make notes of points they want to remember; others use clocks or timers to remember when to take medications.

Other techniques are more ambitious: they seek to improve the patient's cognitive functions by treating the brain like a muscle and relying on the process of neuroplasticity. The underlying theory is that if the patient's brain faces increasingly demanding challenges in daily workouts ("brain games"), the portion of the brain used to meet those challenges will grow—similar to the way muscles develop if they are used in daily workouts.

I regularly played "brain games" during 2014 and 2015. As I gained experience with the games, I became more proficient, and my scores soared. At the same time, however, I did not observe any improvement in my thinking or any increase in my intelligence. In January 2016, the Federal Trade Commission (FTC) announced that the creators and marketers of the Lumosity "brain training" program had agreed to settle FTC charges that they deceived consumers. According to the FTC, Lumosity had made unfounded claims that the program helped users to reduce or delay cognitive impairment.

I meet each week in a group session with a therapist and several other Parkinson's patients. In these sessions, we engage in a variety of activities that require us to use both our brains and our voices. For example, we play a game called "Origins" in which one participant offers two alternative explanations of a familiar phrase or expression (such as "cut and dried") and the other participants try to guess which of the two explanations is correct and which has been invented. In another game, "Fact or Crap," one participant makes a plausible or implausible assertion—for example, that Florence Nightingale, the pioneer of modern nursing, was born in Florence, Italy—and the others guess whether the assertion is "fact" or "crap." Although these activities encourage us to speak louder and more clearly, I have not noticed any improvement in our thinking.

Phyllis Richman: "I don't think that playing [a computer-driven brain game] helps me, except insofar as it gives me a pat on the back and tells me I am doing well."

Joel Havemann: "I doubt that proficiency at a computer-driven brain game has any effect on the brain apart from increasing the patient's performance in playing the game."

My personal experience suggests that exercises targeted at improving certain skills, such as multitasking and concentration, might be effective. After my wife and other members of my family observed—nicely but pointedly—that my automobile driving was deteriorating, I recognized that I had to address the problem. Fortuitously, at a meeting of my support group, I met a psychologist who had been working with Parkinson's patients to assess the effectiveness of computer-based cognitive training. After I told her about my driving problems, she suggested that I try a specific computer-based program. To my surprise, the program focused not on driving but on concentration and multitasking. I found that after I used the program daily for two or three weeks, my driving improved significantly.

Support Groups

Parkinson's can be socially isolating. Many of Parkinson's symptoms—such as tremor, impaired mobility, soft or slurred speech, lack of facial expression, drooling, depression, and anxiety—tend to isolate the patient. These symptoms reduce both the patient's interest in socializing and the patient's capacity to socialize.

Although there is more than one way to overcome Parkinson's isolating effects, I find it very helpful to participate in a support group. Support groups provide opportunities to socialize and to obtain useful information about Parkinson's, such as where to find a voice therapist, an occupational therapist, or a physical therapist who works with Parkinson's patients.

My support group meets roughly twice a month, except for July and August when we are in recess. At each session we meet for two hours or so, usually in the home of one of our members. We occasionally invite an outside speaker (such as a physician, a researcher, a therapist, or a Parkinson's activist) to address us, but more often than not the only speakers at the meeting are members of the group.

My group consists of about 30 patients and partners. Typically 15 or 20 attend each meeting. The group members are all roughly the same age and share, insofar as I can discern, roughly the same socioeconomic status. Because the issues that patients face differ from those that their partners face, we occasionally divide ourselves into two smaller groups to discuss some issues separately.

The severity of the members' symptoms varies considerably. Some are in wheelchairs, some use walkers, and others seem to navigate easily without assistance. Some are very articulate, while others slur their words so much that they are difficult to understand.

A support group meeting serves as a forum for participants to discuss Parkinson's-related issues unselfconsciously and unapologetically. In social settings outside of the group, I am more reluctant to draw attention to Parkinson's-related issues. I don't want to burden others with my health problems, and I don't want to create the impression that Parkinson's is the only subject I care to discuss. Moreover, outsiders are unlikely to know enough about Parkinson's-related issues to discuss them knowledgeably.

I have found participation in a support group to be comforting, informative, and energizing. It is comforting because participants learn that they are not alone; it is informative because patients share their knowledge and experience; and it is energizing because the process of making new friends is uplifting. In addition, if a patient has trouble speaking, a support group is a good place to learn how to address the problem.

A patient or a partner may be able to find an appropriate support group through a local hospital or through the web site of one of the Parkinson's organizations listed in Appendix 3.

• • •

John and Lorrie VerSteeg have found participation in a support group to be very beneficial. The participants in their group include both patients and partners. The patients have a variety of symptoms. Lorrie says that John's current condition alarms some participants whose symptoms are currently less pronounced than his. When asked whether they should be alarmed, Lorrie replies by observing that "everyone is different" and "what John has, others may never encounter."

• • •

Rick Vaughan has adopted a different approach. Rick plays tennis two or three times a week and participates twice a week in a Parkinson's exercise group. Although he has not joined a formally organized support group, he believes that his tennis and exercise groups function as informal support groups.

If you are not inclined to participate in a support group, I suggest giving it a try anyway; you might enjoy it. But if you try it and find it unrewarding, or if you feel uncomfortable in a group for any reason, I would not recommend forcing the issue. Keep your eye on the ball. Support groups are a means to an end; they are not the ultimate objective. There are alternative ways of socializing, obtaining information, and gaining support.

Dan Lewis: "After Vicki and I met with two different support groups, we concluded that we needed to join a group with which we had more in common. We decided to start our own support group. We started with just a few people we had met, and the support group grew from there."

Judy Havemann: "Some support groups attract spouses who complain about patients' behavior, and the support group meetings become complaint sessions. I find that to be counterproductive. Instead of complaining, the spouses should simply do their best and move on."

Glenn Roberts: "I get two principal benefits from my support group. First, it is invaluable as a source of information . . . information about treatment and sources of care. Second, it is a wonderful source of camaraderie, a great place to commiserate without indulging in self-pity."

Kitty Roberts: "If you are a newly diagnosed patient, join a support group for newly diagnosed patients and their partners. Don't join a group for people who are much further along with the disease than you are. If you can't find an existing group that is suitable, start one yourself. Make it happen."

Sarah Boyer: "Join a support group if you can take it. You have to be able to handle the sight of folks who are a lot worse off than you are."

John Boyer: "Support groups are very helpful to partners. The partners who met as a separate group at a support group meeting found a lot of support from the other partners . . . much more so than the patients. I was the only male in the group. A lot of the women are successful in their own right and have active lives and are in quite good shape. But then suddenly they have a tremendous responsibility that disrupts their daily routines, and they don't have anything wrong with them. But they don't get the attention and the sympathy that the patients get—even though their lives are just as disrupted as their spouses' lives. It's almost cathartic for them. . . . It provides an opportunity to share coping mechanisms."

Judy Dodge: "The reason I like it is that everyone has a different story to tell. You recognize that it's not a cut-and-dried illness."

Wilma Hazen: "A support group provides me with emotional support as well as an opportunity to get practical advice from people who have already faced challenges similar to those I am now facing."

Brain Surgery

In 2002 the FDA approved deep brain stimulation (DBS) surgery as a treatment for Parkinson's patients. Although DBS is not suitable for all Parkinson's patients, it does benefit many of them. Currently, approximately 8,000 to 10,000 Parkinson's patients worldwide have DBS surgery each year.

In 2004 or 2005, not long after I was diagnosed with Parkinson's, I heard a radio commercial advertising a local hospital's successful treatment of Parkinson's with DBS surgery. The commercial piqued my curiosity. At my next appointment with my neurologist, I asked him about DBS. He was familiar with the positive results that some patients were getting from it. However, he cautioned that all surgery involves risk, that my symptoms were being adequately treated by medication, and that in all likelihood it would be many years before I would need to consider surgery. The neurologist's advice made sense to me, and for the first four years after I was diagnosed, I relied on medication to manage my symptoms.

By 2008, however, I was disenchanted with all of the medications I was taking, particularly with the side effects, such as dyskinesias and dry mouth. Although brain surgery might seem a risky alternative, I was still intrigued. My neurologist reported recent findings that there were potentially significant benefits from having DBS surgery sooner rather than later. We decided that it made sense to consult a neurosurgeon who was proficient at DBS surgery. I did not hesitate. I called the neurosurgeon's office the next day.

When Joanne and I visited the neurosurgeon, he told us that he would not perform the surgery unless a neurologist that he designated approved it. Fortunately, the designated neurologist was available to see me that day. Arrangements were made for me to have a full-day clinical comprehensive assessment, including an "on/off" medication assessment, neuropsych testing, and an informational meeting. Joanne was also required to complete a detailed questionnaire about me. I must have passed the tests, because the neurosurgeon promptly scheduled me for DBS surgery.

I was excited by the prospect of DBS surgery. In retrospect, I am not sure why I wasn't terrified. Although I recognized that brain surgery was a serious matter and that a favorable outcome was not assured, I had confidence in the surgical team, which was experienced and well known for its DBS prowess.

DBS is typically effective in treating, among other things, slowness of movement, muscle rigidity, tremor, dyskinesias, and gait and mild balance problems that are responsive to levodopa. On the other hand, DBS is not typically effective in treating other Parkinson's symptoms, including cognitive problems, depression, anxiety, speech or swallowing problems, and bladder, bowel, and sexual dysfunction.

The manufacturer of the DBS system warns that DBS is not appropriate, for example, for those who have significant cognitive or psychiatric problems or for those who have a condition requiring them to have many MRI images. The manufacturer also cautions that DBS can trigger or aggravate personality, anxiety, or mood disorders in some patients. In particular, a history of major depression is a risk factor for a significant postoperative mood disorder, even when surgery results in marked improvement in movement.

For DBS surgery, the risks also include the risk of hemorrhage, stroke, and infection. In addition, potential side effects include seizure, infection, memory problems, speech problems, and personality changes. There could be bleeding in the brain when the electrodes are introduced.

My DBS surgery was uneventful. It was performed in two stages in late 2008. The first (in which the electrodes were inserted in my brain) was performed under local anesthesia, so that I was awake throughout the surgery. I was in a reclined position, and my head was placed in a special frame with screws to keep it still. A local anesthetic was applied to the areas where the screws contacted my scalp and to the two locations where the surgeon drilled openings in my skull for the electrodes. The surgery was largely pain-free. I have felt more pain in a dentist's office.

The second surgery was performed several weeks later under general anesthesia. At this stage, the neurosurgeon implanted the neurostimulator (about the size of a stopwatch) under the skin on my chest wall, just below my collarbone. He connected the electrodes to the neurostimulator by making another small opening behind my left ear and then passing wires under the skin of my head, neck, and shoulder. The neurostimulator was powered by a battery with an expected life of about five years. A week or two after the surgery, the neurologist who had cleared me for DBS turned on the neurostimulator and programmed it to function appropriately.

The programming for the neurostimulator can be adjusted without surgery. In my case, the neurologist made such adjustments on several occasions, with no fanfare, at routine office visits. I have reduced my reliance on Parkinson's medications, resulting in a corresponding reduction in dyskinesias. My symptoms have not advanced. I do have two small bumps on the front of my head where the neurosurgeon inserted the electrodes into my brain. Since I am bald, the bumps are easy for others to see. They are not unsightly, however, and are, in my judgment, a very small price to pay for the results of DBS.

Since the installation of the original neurostimulator in 2008, I have returned to the neurosurgeon twice to have him install replacements (one in 2013 and another in 2015) as the power supply declined. Although the first battery lasted for five years, the second lasted for only two years. My neurologist explained that adjustments he had made to the settings for the second neurostimulator caused it to make greater demands on its battery (and to use up the battery's power supply faster) than the first neurostimulator had.

There was no assurance that the battery for the third neurostimulator would last any longer than the second one had, and I did not relish the prospect of having surgery every two years (or less) to replace the device. All surgery involves risk—even if the surgery is relatively minor and even if the risk is small. Accordingly, I elected to have the second neurostimulator replaced by one powered by a *rechargeable* battery. This should last for nine years, after which, because of an FDA requirement, a neurostimulator with a rechargeable battery must be replaced.

I now recharge the battery daily by placing a small recharger on my chest, outside the chest wall where the neurostimulator is located. Recharging takes about 30 minutes. I read, watch television, or make telephone calls during the process. This is a form of multitasking that I can handle. Taking 30 minutes out of the day to recharge my battery is not unpleasant, and on some days it is actually welcome.

I continue to see both neurologists. Like me, they are pleased with the results of the DBS surgery. Occasionally I ask them whether my results are unusual. I know from my support group that some patients have had outcomes not as positive as mine. Yet the neurologists say that my experience is not at all unusual.

As the following summaries indicate, patients have had a range of outcomes with DBS—some quite favorable, and others less so.

• • •

Initially, Dan Lewis's symptoms were mild and limited primarily to the absence of arm swing that Vicki had noticed. However, within a few years, his symptoms expanded to include gait problems. When Dan walked, he shuffled, rather than lifted, his feet. He also had occasional balance problems, becoming unsteady as he navigated around the house or his office. He had episodes of "freezing" in which his feet seemed nailed to the floor. Dan's neurologist prescribed Sinemet. The medication reduced Dan's gait, imbalance, and freezing symptoms, but triggered dyskinesias.

Unhappy with the dyskinesias, Dan had DBS surgery in 2005. The surgery was immediately effective. Dan's dyskinesias and arm-swing, freezing, balance, and gait symptoms were markedly reduced, at least for a few years, and he was able to reduce his daily dosage of medications. However, after the DBS surgery, Dan's speech became increasingly slurred. In recent years, Dan's freezing, balance, and gait problems (which were not expected to be addressed by DBS in the first place) have returned. He no longer drives a car, and he uses a walker to get around by foot.

Dan says that he was very pleased with the results of DBS: "My symptoms receded to where they had been five years earlier. I was able to cut my intake of Sinemet by half, and my dyskinesias were markedly reduced. My symptoms have progressed since then, but I continue to benefit from the five-year boost that I got from DBS."

• • •

Learie Phillip relied on medication to treat Parkinson's until 2006. At about that time, he began to experience severe cramping in his toes and "on/off" fluctuations. In "on" periods, there is enough dopamine in the brain, and the patient can perform many tasks normally or almost normally. At "off" times, insufficient dopamine is present, and the patient becomes very slow and stiff.

Learie's on/off fluctuations became extreme: as the levodopa wore off, and before it was time for the next dose, he could not move. When his neurologist recommended DBS, Learie did not hesitate. The benefits of DBS were palpable: the on/off fluctuations and toe-cramping ceased immediately.

Today Learie is doing well. He exercises every day and participates in a weekly dance class. He has fallen three times, and he now uses a walker to prevent further falls. Although Learie hasn't fallen in the past year or so, he says that the risk of falling is always present and is never far from his mind.

• • •

Anne Davis was very unhappy with the medication she was taking in 2013 (Sinemet). It was instantly effective, but the effectiveness wore off sharply, and she was constantly waiting for the next dose. Anne hated the feeling of being so dependent on medication. Her neurologist explained to her that she was a "poster child" candidate for DBS. The surgery, he said, was perfect for someone who was so responsive to Sinemet and who had such bad "wearing off" periods.

Anne had DBS surgery later in 2013. She does not remember the procedure itself; the doctors gave her a "forgetting drug." However, she recalls that immediately after the surgery, she was "as happy as a bug in a rug." The day of her DBS surgery "was the best day of my life," she explains. Her medication was immediately cut in half. Her symptoms were less pronounced. She could walk much more easily.

Anne says that her personality changed immediately after her surgery. Before DBS, she felt terrible anxiety—particularly when driving. She was anxious about driving off the road or into a truck. After her DBS surgery, it was just the opposite. Far from being anxious while driving, Anne became overconfident. "I was jumping around," she says.

According to Anne, she took on the personality of a 14-year-old. "I was a crazy person." She says that the period of erratic behavior subsided after the first year and eventually ended only because of the passage of time. "My husband bore the brunt of it," she acknowledges.

Anne now feels great. Whereas she had "lost [her] smile" before the DBS surgery, people now tell her that she has a beautiful smile.

Anne still has some Parkinson's symptoms. She has fainting spells and periods when she feels compelled to walk. She has some difficulty sleeping, and she has a tremor that she didn't have pre-

viously. On the whole, however, Anne believes that DBS was great
for her.

Anne's chief concern is cognitive impairment. Before she had
DBS surgery, she could complete rather easily the crossword puzzles in *The Washington Post*. Those puzzles are far more difficult
for her now. She also played computer-driven "brain games" both
before and after her DBS; her scores are now significantly lower
than they were before the surgery. She attributes the cognitive decline to her DBS surgery.

• • •

Although Phyllis Richman never had a tremor, she began to be
plagued by dyskinesias during 2009. Unhappy with this problem, Phyllis elected to have DBS surgery in 2013. The surgery suc-
ceeded in completely eliminating the dyskinesias, but left Phyllis
with little energy, and she attributes her erratic exercise habits in
recent months to the surgery's effect on her vigor.

• • •

John VerSteeg had DBS surgery in May of 2004. In 2011 John and
Lorrie noticed a lesion on the left side of his head where the DBS
lead wire entered. John had the lesion removed in November 2012,
but nothing more was done at that time. In May 2013, John's newly
assigned neurosurgeon found that the lead wire had broken and
removed it. This neurosurgeon also found that the lesion was can-
cerous and that John had developed a staph infection. The neurosurgeon recommended that the DBS system be replaced, but John
and Lorrie had had enough. As Lorrie puts it, "Overall we feel John
is better without the system, but only God knows for sure."

John's symptoms have advanced slowly, but markedly, over the
past 25 years. His tremors have become much more severe; his
muscles have become more rigid; he cannot write legibly; he has
great difficulty walking; and his cognitive abilities have declined.

Balance is also a problem for John; his upper body leans to the
left, causing him to fall often. When his medications are not working or have worn off, he has episodes of freezing. John now gets
around by using a walker or a wheelchair. At home, when his legs

are freezing, or when he feels unsteady on his feet, he resorts to crawling.

John has difficulty bathing and dressing. Eating is becoming more and more difficult; his tremors often make it impossible for him to hold utensils. John also suffers from mild depression and sleeps a lot.

• • •

Larry Baskir was 70 years old when he was diagnosed with Parkinson's. He had DBS surgery five years later. At age 75, Larry was older than most DBS patients, and, unlike most who opt for the surgery, he had significant nonmovement symptoms, including occasional hallucinations, anxiety, cognitive difficulties, and low blood pressure.

Before deciding to proceed with DBS, Larry and his wife, Marna, consulted a number of neurologists and neurosurgeons. All of them gave essentially the same advice: that DBS surgery was appropriate. Although the couple was told that the surgery would not ameliorate Larry's nonmovement symptoms, no one suggested that the surgery was inadvisable.

Larry and Marna also discussed DBS surgery with members of their support group. Several members had recently undergone the surgery, and several others were actively considering it. Those who had recently been operated on were pleased with the results, and those who were considering the surgery were optimistic. Encouraged by these discussions, Larry and Marna decided to proceed with DBS surgery. Although they did not expect the surgery to reduce Larry's hallucinations or his anxiety or cognitive problems, neither did they expect the surgery to aggravate them. Based on the advice they had obtained, Larry and Marna believed that their expectations regarding the outcome of the surgery were reasonable.

The outcome differed markedly from what Larry and Marna expected, however. During the first few months following the surgery, Larry was agitated and psychotic. Initially he did not understand why he was in the hospital and thought he was imprisoned there. Larry talked to his doctor about trying to escape.

The hospital gave Larry a variety of drugs to calm him down, put mittens on his hands to prevent him from tearing out the tubes and wires attached to him, and applied restraints to keep him from getting out of bed. Larry's neurostimulator also was turned off, but that did not improve his condition.

After consulting a number of psychiatrists and neurologists, Marna found a geriatrician (a physician who specializes in caring for older people) with substantial experience in treating agitated patients. This doctor suggested that creating a more familiar environment for Larry at the hospital would reduce his agitation.

Following the geriatrician's recommendations, Marna arranged for a reclining chair in Larry's hospital room for him to sit in during the day, hung pictures of their grandchildren on the walls, brought in a radio and a CD player so that Larry could listen to his favorite music, and arranged for lamps to illuminate the hospital room with light that was warmer than the light cast by the hospital's overhead lights. These measures promptly reduced Larry's agitation.

Marna also urged the hospital to find a cure for Larry's psychosis. The only remedy appeared to be strong antipsychotic drugs, which did not become effective immediately and required careful supervision by a psychiatrist. The hospital put Larry on a regimen of antipsychotic drugs under the supervision of the hospital's psychiatric department.

Gradually, over more than a month, Larry's agitation disappeared and the psychosis subsided. Once he calmed down and was communicative, he was ready to go home. At home, Larry continued to take the antipsychotic drugs under the supervision of a psychiatrist. The drugs were gradually reduced and were eliminated after another month.

Larry's neurologist also recommended that the DBS neurostimulator be turned on under careful monitoring in a hospital setting. Although turning on the neurostimulator did not affect Larry's gait or balance, it did enable him to cut in half his daily dose of Sinemet. Larry had been having pronounced dyskinesias, but the dyskinesias virtually disappeared after he reduced his dosage of Sinemet.

Larry is at home now. However, for much of the day, he is tired: he is largely inactive, and he prefers to keep his eyes closed. Although Larry's demeanor during these periods might suggest that he is "out of it," Marna says that he is very much aware of what is going on. Moreover, Larry is back to normal during the early evening hours (5:00 p.m. to 10:00 p.m.), when he and Marna go out to dinner, visit with friends, and attend concerts, as they did prior to the surgery.

Based on what they have learned since the surgery, Larry and Marna now believe that Larry was not a strong candidate for DBS and that his relatively advanced age and hallucinations were warning signs that probably should have excluded him.

Before making a decision regarding DBS, a patient should go through a very careful evaluation at a medical center with considerable experience with DBS. An NIH report concludes:

> Although most individuals still need to take medication after undergoing DBS, many people with Parkinson's disease experience considerable reduction of their motor symptoms and are able to reduce their medications. The amount of reduction varies but [the medications] can be considerably reduced in most individuals, and can lead to a significant improvement in side effects. . . . DBS does not improve cognitive symptoms in PD and indeed may worsen them, so it is not generally used if there are signs of dementia. DBS changes the brain firing pattern but does not slow the progression of the neurodegeneration. (National Institute of Neurological Disorders and Stroke, "NINDS Deep Brain Stimulation for Parkinson's Disease Information Page")

Marna Tucker: "If we had known then what we know now, I am not sure that we would have chosen to have DBS surgery."

Stress Management

Stress often aggravates Parkinson's symptoms, at least temporarily. For example, tremors (both those that are caused by Parkinson's and those that are not) become more pronounced when the individual is under stress. Similarly, slowness and gait problems may worsen. Stress also contributes to a number of illnesses and addictions, such as high blood pressure, strokes, heart disease, obesity, cigarette and drug addiction, and alcoholism.

A dopamine deficiency impairs a patient's ability to cope with stress. That is because the body needs adrenaline to cope with stress, and the body uses dopamine to produce adrenaline.

I rely on a variety of techniques to cope with or reduce stress: I have withdrawn from the stressful aspects of law practice. I don't try to conceal my disease. I exercise regularly. I socialize with friends. I participate in support group meetings. I try to maintain a positive attitude. And I try to avoid stressful situations by, for example, budgeting plenty of time for an appointment or meeting and arriving at a doctor's office well before the appointment time, at a movie theater well before the start time, and at a train station or airport well before the scheduled departure.

Another strategy for stress reduction is to practice a discipline such as tai chi, yoga, or meditation in which controlled breathing is taught. Although I have not tried one of these disciplines myself, some patients have found them helpful for controlling stress. In addition, cognitive-behavioral therapy with a psychologist can help the patient deal with stress, as well as with depression and anxiety issues.

Diet

To my knowledge, no food or diet has been proven to prevent or slow the advance of Parkinson's. However, a healthy diet with plenty of water can help manage some of Parkinson's symptoms, such as constipation, and help maintain bone strength (reducing the risk of a fracture in the event of a fall). A healthy diet includes plenty of grain products, bran cereals, fruits and vegetables, and foods low in fat.

Because the brain's absorption of levodopa can be slowed by a high-protein meal, some patients limit the protein they consume, eating most of their protein in the evening and not much at breakfast or lunch. My neurologist tells me, however, that I should consume a minimum of about 60 grams of protein a day.

Many patients report that their diet does not affect their movement function. That includes me. I have not altered my consumption of protein, and this practice has not had any adverse consequence that I can discern. I would not adopt a low-protein diet without conferring with my doctor.

Judy Havemann: "[Joel] believed firmly that eating too much protein inhibited the effects of the medicine he was taking. So he used to cut up all this fruit. He practically lived on fruit. It's amazing that he hasn't become a tree with leaves. He used to eat this vast amount of fruit during the day and one meal at night where he had some protein and that was always very limited. I think that probably helped. Whether that was essential to being able to work for almost 20 years after he was diagnosed, I don't know, but it seemed as if it was."

Complementary Therapies

Because traditional therapies do not cure Parkinson's or completely eliminate all of its symptoms, some patients use complementary therapies together with traditional ones.

I am not aware of any scientific evidence that any complementary therapy slows, stops, or reverses Parkinson's or its symptoms. There are many complementary therapies, however, and different ones might work for different people.

Three cautions. First, a complementary therapy is just that. It complements, rather than replaces, a traditional therapy. Second, in my judgment, a complementary therapy (or any therapy for that matter) should be tried only after consulting a qualified neu-rologist. For example, although a low-protein diet might help the body to use levodopa and carbidopa efficiently, the patient should not adopt such a diet without checking with his or her doctor first. Third, I cannot vouch for the effectiveness or safety of *any* complementary therapy; I have not tried any of them.

Massage. Massage has been reported to provide temporary symptomatic relief to Parkinson's patients. The reported benefits include reduced rigidity, tremor, and muscle tension, improved sleep, increased stamina, reduced anxiety, and greater relaxation. Massage has also been said to reduce pain, to improve movement and flexibility, and to help with constipation.

Bert King: "My neurologist recommended massage, and I have found massage to be very beneficial. It helps to loosen up my muscles. Massage complements the stretching that is also part of my regular exercise program. I find that stretching and massage are, together, more effective at loosening up my muscles than is stretching alone.

"You need to get massage regularly, and that can be costly. To keep my costs down, I use electrical equipment rather than a professional masseur. The electrical equipment is very effective, but it is less flexible than a professional masseur."

Antioxidants, supplements, and vitamins. Antioxidants, such as Vitamins C and E, have been studied to see if they protect neurons. However, these studies have not yet demonstrated that either vitamin has a neuroprotective role. The results of studies on other vitamins and supplements are mixed. For example, a large clinical trial demonstrated that Coenzyme Q10 was not helpful to Parkinson's patients.

My internist recommended that I take a daily dose of Vitamin D, and I do so. Parkinson's patients often have low levels of Vitamin D, and taking the vitamin as a supplement can help prevent osteoporosis, which is of particular concern to Parkinson's patients.

• • •

One patient I interviewed takes an array of supplements, including multivitamins, creatine, omega-3, and antioxidants. The patient does not do this casually. Rather, the patient follows the recommendations of a physician who is a pain management specialist. The physician has carefully layered the supplements to distinguish those that are helpful from those that are not. The doctor checks the patient's blood counts every three months and adjusts the supplements as and when appropriate.

Herbal medicine. Herbal medicine relies on compounds made from plants or plant components. For example, gingko is said to be an antioxidant that improves blood flow to the brain and helps to deliver dopamine. These compounds are not regulated by the FDA, however, and many are imported from countries where there is no quality control. In addition, the compounds are potentially harmful and may interact with medications that the patient is taking.

Hypnosis. Hypnosis can put a patient in a state of deep relaxation. There are anecdotal reports that this has helped some people to control pain and others to cope with sleep disorders and depression. However, I am not aware of any clinical proof of benefits to Parkinson's patients.

Phyllis Richman: "Although the hypnotist had not previously tried to cure freezing problems, I was optimistic, and the hypnotist was willing to give it a try. He gave me a self-hypnosis tape and several meditation tapes. The meditation tapes were relaxing, but I am not sufficiently visual to allow the hypnosis to work. Hypnosis might work for someone who is more visual than I am, but for now at least hypnosis is not for me."

Acupuncture. Acupuncture calls for the insertion of hair-like needles at certain points on the body to correct any imbalance in the flow of energy. I am not aware of any study that makes a convincing case for the effectiveness of acupuncture for Parkinson's disease. Research is now under way, however, to determine if acupuncture can help patients cope with fatigue. Fatigue affects approximately half of all Parkinson's patients, and traditional medications do not offer much help.

Scott Kragie: "Acupuncture provided me with what was at most temporary relief from muscular aches and pains."

Chuck Linderman: "I did not find acupuncture to be at all effective in relieving pain."

Barriers to Access

Unfortunately, not all patients have access to therapies that treat Parkinson's effectively. Socioeconomic, geographic, and other barriers prevent many patients from getting the help they need.

Scott Kragie: "Without money, Parkinson's is a different disease."

Socioeconomic status. Although I did not conduct a sufficient number of interviews to allow firm conclusions about the effect of socioeconomic status, it does seem that socioeconomic factors help to explain why many patients do not have access to (or do not take advantage of) effective Parkinson's therapies.

Health care cost. The high cost of health care prevents many patients from taking advantage of effective therapies. This is clearly so for those who do not have health insurance. Even after the enactment of the Affordable Care Act, approximately 30 million Americans went without health insurance for all of 2014. Millions more were uninsured for part of the year.

Moreover, even for those Americans who have health insurance coverage, the cost of care can be a barrier. Although an individual might be covered by an employer-sponsored health plan or a governmental health plan (such as Medicare), coverage by those plans is not costless to the insured. Even if a patient can afford to bear the additional health care costs that Parkinson's entails, the disease may require the patient to use financial resources that the patient had set aside for some other purpose (for retirement income, for example).

Other costs. Even the most comprehensive health care plans do not cover all additional costs, such as gym membership dues incurred to maintain physical fitness. Although some patients can afford to bear those costs, many cannot.

Ignorance. Patients with a low socioeconomic status may mistakenly believe that slowness and tremor are the normal consequences of aging or that their symptoms must become more severe before they can get treatment. Of course, other patients may share this misunderstanding, but perhaps not to the same extent.

Other health conditions. Some low-income patients have other chronic health conditions and assign their Parkinson's symptoms a lower priority than their other symptoms. Some are alcoholic, and they (or their physicians) may mistakenly dismiss their Parkinson's symptoms as symptoms of alcohol abuse.

Mistrust. There are numerous studies indicating that low-income patients (and low-income African-Americans in particular) are more likely than other patients to mistrust physicians. Someone who mistrusts physicians in general is less likely to consult a neurologist who can diagnose and treat Parkinson's.

Discomfort. Patients who are unaccustomed to dealing with medical specialists may be reluctant to consult them. By contrast, a patient with a higher socioeconomic status may have little discomfort in relating to a medical specialist, and may even regard the physician as a peer. In some cases, the specialist may be the patient's neighbor, friend, or relative.

Fear of discovery. Some low-income patients are in the United States unlawfully. Fear of being discovered may discourage these patients from seeking medical help.

Referrals. Physicians may be less likely to refer a patient with a lower socioeconomic status to a specialist—perhaps because the patient is less likely to ask for (or to insist on) a referral. Moreover, when a physician does refer a patient with a lower socioeconomic status to a specialist, the patient may be less likely than others to follow up.

Giving up. I spoke to a physical therapist who said, "It's not because [low-income patients] don't have Parkinson's. It's because they give up. . . . If you think it's difficult for you to fight Parkinson's with all the resources you have access to, try to imagine how difficult it is for them. Many just give up."

Complexity of the system. Because of difficulties in navigating the U.S. health care system, a patient who is educated, English-speaking, and engaged will probably receive better treatment for Parkinson's than will an uneducated, non-English-speaking, or unengaged patient. Furthermore, as illustrated by a number of the cases recounted in this book, patients who are friends, relatives, or neighbors of physicians can more easily navigate the system than those without such connections.

Geography. Patients residing near major medical centers can gain access to the therapies they need more readily than patients residing elsewhere. Patients who live near major medical centers can draw upon the experience and expertise of neurologists, neurosurgeons, and other professionals, and benefit from the support of other patients and their partners. Although there are advantages to living in more isolated parts of the country, patients in those areas often lack access to medical expertise.

• • •

Living with Parkinson's far from a major medical center can be like running a marathon without having trained for it. As residents of Kalamazoo County, Michigan (approximate population

256,000), John and Lorrie VerSteeg confront challenges that people residing in larger metropolitan areas do not have to face.

It has been difficult for John to find a neurologist in Kalamazoo with expertise in Parkinson's. Although John had DBS surgery in Kalamazoo, he was not able to find a neurologist there to adjust the device that the surgeon implanted. Accordingly, John traveled about 250 miles to the Cleveland Clinic in Cleveland, where a neurologist made the necessary adjustments.

Lorrie now drives John twice a year to the Cleveland Clinic, a 10-hour round trip. Diagnosed with Parkinson's disease nearly 25 years ago, John is not in a condition to help with the driving. Lorrie handles the semiannual drive without complaint, but it is not easy.

John and Lorrie are not alone. They participate in a support group in Kalamazoo, and they report that other Parkinson's patients and partners in the group regularly make similar trips from Kalamazoo to Ann Arbor, Detroit, or Grand Rapids.

• • •

Pete and Maggie Riehm try to take advantage of resources available to those in the Washington, DC–Baltimore area, including access to the National Institutes of Health, Georgetown University, Johns Hopkins, the University of Maryland, at least one large private practice specializing in Parkinson's, the Parkinson's Foundation of the National Capital Area, and the numerous panel discussions, support groups, exercise groups, and seminars that these institutions sponsor or foster.

Pete and Maggie learned how lucky they were when, in 2010, they went on a Caribbean cruise sponsored by a Parkinson's organization in the Sarasota, Florida, area. Many of the people on the cruise did not live near a major medical center and signed up for the cruise in order to obtain the information and emotional support that Pete and Maggie find routinely available.

• • •

Sandra Ridinger has a different take on this issue. A 74-year-old widow, Sandra lives in Christiansburg (population 21,000), a small town in rural southern Virginia, about 35 miles outside of Roanoke. Sandra believes, quite firmly, that insofar as her Parkinson's disease is concerned, living in Christiansburg is an advantage, not a disadvantage.

In Christiansburg, Sandra is part of a tight-knit group of women who function, for Sandra, largely in the same way as a conventional Parkinson's support group. The women are extremely supportive of one another, and, as Sandra puts it, they "do everything together."

I say that Sandra's group functions *largely* in the same way as a Parkinson's support group because the other members are not patients or partners. This makes a difference, as Sandra recognizes. For example, when Sandra has a freezing episode, as she does from time to time, her friends encourage her, but without the understanding that another patient would have of how difficult it is for Sandra to overcome the feeling that her feet are glued to the floor. Sandra says that she feels as though she is the only person in the world who has to endure freezing.

Although Sandra lives alone, she is also supported by her family: two of her three sisters live in Christiansburg, and her children and some of her grandchildren live in nearby Roanoke.

Sandra was diagnosed in 2003. She noticed a tremor in the pinky of her left hand, and her handwriting had become remarkably small, virtually illegible. Sandra consulted her internist in Christiansburg about her symptoms, and he referred her to a neurologist in Roanoke who diagnosed her.

Today, Sandra no longer has a tremor, and her handwriting is back to normal. Her principal symptoms are freezing and illusions. Sandra is anxious about the future. She is keenly aware that her symptoms could, and probably will, change.

Maggie Riehm: "We are very lucky living where we do . . . in the Silicon Valley of medical research [suburban Washington, DC]."

No spouse or domestic partner. A spouse or domestic partner often is the first to spot the patient's symptoms and to encourage evaluation by a doctor. An individual with no spouse or domestic partner (or other close family member) is less likely to seek health care promptly.

Confusion or denial. Although they don't necessarily realize it, some patients do not take advantage of all of the therapies available to them. For example, an individual who attributes Parkinson's symptoms to old age rather than to disease is less likely to receive appropriate therapies.

Attitude

I believe my attitude serves me well in my battle against Parkinson's. Three firm beliefs shape my attitude. First, I believe that I have no reason to feel sorry for myself. I have enjoyed more than my share of good luck. In a world in which so many people suffer, I have no reason to expect to be exempt from Parkinson's or any other chronic disease. Second, I believe that I am not required to accept whatever the disease imposes on me. I have the capacity to manage Parkinson's symptoms. Third, I believe that although Parkinson's deprives me of opportunities, it also gives me opportunities, including the chance to show what I am and who I am.

Other Parkinson's patients have adopted similar attitudes— often under circumstances far more difficult than mine. As the following paragraphs show, attitude makes a big difference.

• • •

Following his diagnosis in 1989, Joel Havemann continued to work for nearly 20 years. Joel elected to have DBS surgery in 2004, and he describes the impact of the surgery as "huge." The severity of his symptoms immediately declined. Joel's tremors became less pronounced; his dyskinesias were much reduced; and he became much less reliant on medication.

More recently, in 2013, Joel's vision and cognitive abilities began to decline. Now he can read only with great difficulty. He often has trouble formulating his thoughts, and sometimes is unable to complete a sentence that he has started. Today, although Joel wants to be a helpful and contributing member of his family, and although he wants to do things for other people, he can't drive, he can't walk without a walker, and his voice is very difficult to understand over the telephone. Notwithstanding all of this, Joel persists. He remains positive and well informed.

When asked to explain how Joel remains upbeat in such difficult circumstances, his wife, Judy, points to his fundamentally positive personality. She says that Joel has always been optimistic and cheerful, never negative or gloomy.

Judy Havemann: "It does seem as if the [Parkinson's patient] has quite a bit of control over how it actually goes, and so people who are careful about diet, and careful about exercise, and careful about those things that you actually have control over can actually slow down the disease."

• • •

Until his death in 2014, Michael Rosenbush was a fighter. In his earliest years, he learned the importance of fighting. Although 80 members of his family perished in the Holocaust, Michael and his parents survived. He could recall being carried by his parents as they escaped the Nazis on a route that took them through Siberia. It was a lesson that Michael could not and did not forget. When he was diagnosed with Parkinson's, he was determined to fight it, and he did. He did not just go through the motions. He exercised. He sang. He participated in a support group.

• • •

Parkinson's is hardly the only challenge that Sarah Boyer has faced in recent years. Since 2003, Sarah has been treated for depression, broken her clavicle and two ribs as a result of a fall, had knee replacement surgery, had adrenal failure (Addison's disease), and developed (and been treated for) arthritis in her spine.

To top it off, in March 2013, Sarah was diagnosed with breast cancer. She went through surgery, radiation, and chemotherapy. Sarah says with a laugh that now that she has cancer, she is "over" Parkinson's and "into" cancer. She reports that she is now doing well, and a recent bone scan showed no trace of cancer.

Sarah considers herself lucky. She is doing very well, all things considered. As Sarah puts it, she is "hanging in there."

Joanne Vine: "Don't give in. Exercise. Be tenacious. The future course of the disease may depend on luck, but good luck often comes to those who work hard."

Judy Havemann: "Attitude toward the disease has an impact. People who give up or who say I am out of here and I'm going to quit my job, those who say I'm too sick to work and I can't function any more—they *are* too sick to work, and they *can't* function any more. By contrast, those who have the attitude that I am going to keep going as long as I can, and that I'm going to fight this as long as I can and live as normal a life as I can, it does seem to me that it helps."

Rick Vaughan: "Be positive and stay active. When combined with appropriate medications and a little luck, these constitute the four factors that most affect Parkinson's patients.

"To a large extent, attitude and activity are the factors a patient can control."

Bert King: "Originally, Parkinson's made me feel as though I had drawn the short straw. But now I realize that everyone is carrying baggage. You just have to maintain the right attitude. Living with Parkinson's is like wrestling a lion. You have to fight it. You have to push yourself. It's the only way you are going to get results. You can't give up."

Activism

When asked what word best describes his attitude toward Parkinson's, Dan Lewis does not hesitate. He says "defiance." When Dan says "defiance," he means it. Dan battles Parkinson's daily on

his own behalf, on behalf of Parkinson's patients in his community, and on behalf of Parkinson's patients throughout the United
States.

Dan exercises every day. He exercises with a Parkinson's group
three times a week, with an aerobics class twice a week, and with
a personal trainer twice a week; he has two sessions a week with
a voice therapist; and he participates in a Parkinson's singing
group once a week.

Dan and his wife, Vicki, are the leaders of a support group they
started in 2005. Always optimistic, constructive, energetic, and
generous, they host and organize meetings and outings and set
the agenda for each meeting.

Dan serves on the board of directors of the Parkinson's Foundation of the National Capital Area. He was the board chairman
from 2012 until 2014. A forceful and energetic advocate for federal funding for Parkinson's research, he has served on the board
of directors of the Parkinson's Action Network.

For Dan, activism is a form of therapy. His defiant stance dem-
onstrates that Parkinson's patients need not be muzzled by the
disease. By acting as advocates for other patients in the community and throughout the country, they can improve their own
health as well as the health of other Parkinson's patients.

• • •

In San Diego, Parkinson's patients and their families and friends
have established a nonprofit organization called Summit for Stem
Cell. The organization's mission is to obtain the funding required
to support nonembryonic stem cell research for the treatment of
Parkinson's disease now being conducted in San Diego by researchers at The Scripps Research Institute and clinicians at Scripps
Clinic (see Chapter 8). Summit for Stem Cell raises funds through
hikes, walks, lab tours, presentations, and pledges by individuals
and corporations.

In July 2016, the Scripps researchers were awarded a grant of
nearly $2.4 million by the California Institute for Regenerative
Medicine (CIRM), a state agency formed in 2004 when California voters approved Proposition 71, the California Stem Cell Re-

search and Cures Initiative. The grant is expected to enable the Scripps researchers to get near the point where they can seek FDA approval to launch clinical trials.

Cassandra Peters: "In the months following my diagnosis with Parkinson's, I would sit for hours in a dark room and say, 'Why? Why me?'

"Now I know the answer. My disease has a purpose. I am one of the patients who will participate in a research project that will determine whether Parkinson's can be treated with nonembryonic stem cells."

CHAPTER 8

Tomorrow's Therapies

ADVANCES IN SCIENCE and medicine during the past 50 years have transformed what it means to have Parkinson's disease. As mentioned in the preceding chapter, the introduction of levodopa in 1967 significantly reduced the severity of the disease's symptoms and dramatically increased the life expectancy of Parkinson's patients. Although it is impossible to predict with confidence what the future will bring, the rate of scientific and medical advance appears to be accelerating. The advances of the next 10 or 20 years could far surpass the very substantial advances of the past 50 years.

The therapies described in this chapter are *potential* therapies. They are still being developed and have not yet received FDA approval. Moreover, other potential new therapies are in the pipeline. The therapies described in this chapter illustrate why today's newly diagnosed Parkinson's patients can hope that a cure for the disease will one day be available to them.

Stem Cell Therapy

Scientists are attempting to use stem cells to produce healthy dopamine-producing neurons that would replace Parkinson's patients' missing neurons. Although the use of *embryonic* stem cells to solve medical problems has been controversial, those controversies can now be avoided by using *nonembryonic stem cells.*

Until relatively recently, scientists worked with only two types of stem cells: embryonic and adult. Embryonic stem cells derive from embryos and can become all cell types—that is, they are "pluripotent." By contrast, adult stem cells are not pluripotent; they can develop only into cell types matching their tissue or organ of origin. Adult stem cells have been identified in many tissues and organs, including brain, bone marrow, skin, teeth, and gut.

In 2007 researchers in Japan discovered that some specialized adult cells could be "reprogrammed" to achieve an embryonic-like state. This new cell is called an induced pluripotent stem cell, or an IPS cell. IPS cells are created by converting a mature adult cell, such as a skin cell, into an embryonic-like state. The IPS cells can then be converted into other cell types.

Now scientists are planning to use IPS cells to create dopamine-producing neurons. They would do this by obtaining specialized adult cells (skin cells, for example) and converting those adult cells into IPS cells. The researchers would then convert the new IPS cells into dopamine-producing neurons, which could be implanted in the brains of Parkinson's patients.

In San Diego, Scripps Clinic and The Scripps Research Institute have begun the research phase of a proposed clinical trial for a *patient-specific* stem cell therapy that would use IPS cells derived from skin cells taken from the Parkinson's patients themselves. Because the patient's own skin cells are used to create the IPS cells and the dopamine-producing neurons, the patient is not expected to reject the implanted neurons. The goal is for the new neurons to produce enough dopamine to alleviate Parkinson's movement symptoms.

The Scripps researchers have already used IPS cells derived from Parkinson's patients to create dopamine-producing neurons. They have also used dopamine-producing neurons to reverse the pathology of Parkinson's disease in rodents. The proposed clinical trial is the next step.

Similar research is taking place at the Harvard Stem Cell Institute (HSCI). In March 2015, HSCI researchers announced that they had used the IPS cells of a primate to treat the primate's Parkinson's disease. The researchers reported that dopamine-producing neurons derived from the primate's own skin cells survived for more than two years after implantation and significantly reduced the animal's Parkinson's symptoms.

Originally, the HSCI experiments were conducted using neurons derived from embryonic stem cells, which required the researchers to use immunosuppressive drugs (drugs that suppress the reaction of the body's immune system to the presence of foreign matter in the body). These experiments did not produce results as positive as those obtained by using the primate's own IPS cells.

The primate that received dopamine-producing neurons derived from its own skin cells did not require immunosuppression. Although the researchers described this as an important step toward treating Parkinson's, the positive results were seen in only one animal, and stem cell treatments for Parkinson's are still in the early stages of development.

Researchers at the Center for iPS Cell Research and Applications at Kyoto University and researchers at the International Stem Cell Corporation, working separately, also have announced plans to begin clinical studies of somewhat different cell replacement therapies that use human IPS cells to treat Parkinson's.

Immunotherapy

Since researchers have suspected for some time that the accumulation of alpha-synuclein protein causes, or helps to cause, Parkinson's, it is not surprising that some are considering whether halting the accumulation of alpha-synuclein might be helpful.

Efforts are under way to use immunotherapy for this purpose. Immunotherapy is a biological therapy that uses substances to stimulate or suppress the body's immune system.

Several biotech companies are seeking to develop vaccines that would prompt the body's own immune system to attack the bad protein—as if it were a virus or bacteria. Any such vaccines are years away, however. The science is challenging, and a new vaccine must satisfy FDA requirements before it can be made publicly available.

Other Therapies

Nilotinib. In May 2013, researchers at Georgetown University Medical Center announced that they had used tiny doses of a leukemia drug called nilotinib to halt the accumulation of alpha-synuclein in the brains of mice. Georgetown has launched a Phase I clinical trial to determine the appropriate dosage and whether the drug hits the appropriate target in humans.

Although encouraging, the initial study of nilotinib as a drug for Parkinson's was relatively small. Moreover, it was an open study: both doctors and patients knew they were testing the drug. A larger, more robust study is required to establish nilotinib's effectiveness. If the results of the Phase I study are positive, the next step will be a Phase II, multi-site, double-blind, placebo-controlled clinical trial.

In a placebo-controlled trial, some participants receive the new drug while others receive a placebo (a pill that contains no medication). "Double-blind" means that neither the patients nor the doctors who assess the results know who received the new drug and who received the placebo. Multi-site means that the trial is conducted at different locations and run by different investigators, further supporting the trial's objectivity.

In most clinical trials of new drugs for Parkinson's disease, some of the patients who have been given the placebo report that it ameliorated their Parkinson's symptoms. There are a number of possible reasons for this "placebo effect," one of which may be an increase in the patient's dopamine level. Experts say that when a patient participates in a trial of a new drug and anticipates a positive effect, the dopamine level in the brain often increases, improving the patient's symptoms. Further study is required to understand the placebo effect and its impact on clinical trials of new Parkinson's drugs.

Peptide. A study led by the University of Bath in the United Kingdom suggests that a peptide—a chain of amino acids—may slow the progression of Parkinson's. Dr. Jody Mason, from the university's Department of Biology & Biochemistry, explained:

> If you think of the misshapen α-synuclein proteins as Lego bricks which stack to form a tower, our peptide acts like a smooth brick that sticks to the α-synuclein and stops the tower from growing any bigger.
>
> This research is in the early stages, but the results so far are very encouraging. We still need to overcome many obstacles before this can be developed into a drug treatment, but these findings could herald a new approach to treating Parkinson's. (Parkinson's UK Press Release, "Sticky Protein Hails New Approach for Treating Parkinson's," 2015.)

Chloroquine and amodiaquine. In 2015 an international team of scientists from Harvard Medical School, McLean Hospital, and Singapore's Nanyang Technological University announced that two popular antimalaria drugs—chloroquine and amodiaquine—could activate a class of proteins that alleviate the symptoms of Parkinson's disease. When activated, these proteins—called NURR1—help the brain to produce, maintain, and protect dopamine neurons.

The announcement of the drugs' apparent effectiveness was based on laboratory tests with rodents. The scientists say that they are trying to design better drugs for Parkinson's by modifying chloroquine and amodiaquine and hope to conduct clinical trials soon.

The safety of taking these drugs for an extended period of time must also be examined. Even healthy people who take these drugs for short periods sometimes develop serious side effects. However, since the drugs have already been approved for the treatment of malaria, the required testing for the treatment of Parkinson's may not be as onerous as it otherwise would be.

Focused ultrasound. University of Virginia and University of Maryland researchers have started using MRI-guided focused ultrasound to destroy the brain cells that interfere with a Parkinson's patient's ability to control body movements. The treatments are part of studies of some 40 patients assessing the feasibility, safety, and preliminary efficacy of focused ultrasound treatments for Parkinson's disease. Studies are being conducted in Canada and Korea as well.

Like focused ultrasound, DBS (discussed in detail earlier) targets specific cells in the brain. DBS, however, requires a hole to be cut in the patient's head so an electrode can be placed in the brain. By contrast, focused ultrasound requires no cutting or insertion of a foreign body. Instead, ultrasound waves are directed through the patient's skull. The waves provide energy low enough to avoid damaging the brain but high enough so that, when the waves meet at a single point, their combined energy creates enough heat to kill the target cells. Experts caution, however, that additional research is required to determine the effectiveness and value of focused ultrasound.

Telemedicine

In the not-too-distant future, U.S. patients with neurological conditions may be able to obtain care in their homes through web-based video conferencing, often referred to as "telemedicine." Physicians can use video conferencing to observe how patients are doing without touching them. A patient's tremor and gait, for example, can be evaluated remotely.

Parkinson's patients in remote locations may be particularly well-suited for such care. However, there are legal, financial, and other barriers to be overcome before telemedicine is widely used. Providing care across state lines is problematic, and restrictions on Medicare coverage also can be a barrier.

CHAPTER 9

Questions

IF YOU ARE a newly diagnosed patient, you probably have questions for your neurologist about the disease and its likely impact on your life. Because you may find it difficult to remember all of your questions, it might help to keep a notebook handy and to jot down your questions as they occur to you. Bring the notebook to your appointments with your neurologist. The following questions are illustrative:

- How certain are you that I have Parkinson's? Why?
- What else could it be?
- Should I get a second opinion?
- Are you a movement disorders specialist? If not, should I see one?
- Should I get a DaTscan test?
- What other professionals should I consult? Should I get occupational therapy, physical therapy, cognitive therapy, and/or speech therapy? If so, can you recommend a therapist?
- What should I tell my family and friends?
- What should I tell my employer?

- May I continue to work?
- May I continue to drive?
- What are my treatment options? What are the pros and cons of each?
- Will it affect my sex life? What can I do about it?
- Do my medications have potential side effects? What are they?
- What about my diet? What should I emphasize or avoid?
- What type(s) of physical exercise do you recommend?
- Are others in my family at risk?

You might bring someone to your initial appointments with the neurologist to record the answers. You might want to update your questions periodically; as you gain more experience, you will learn more about Parkinson's, but you will also have more questions about the disease.

CHAPTER 10

The Bell Lap

WHEN THE LEADER of a distance race at a track meet begins the final lap, a bell rings. This is the bell lap. The bell tells the competitors that if they are going to make a move, they must do so before it is too late. After the race ends, a competitor does not benefit from any energy that he or she has saved.

Like the bell at a track meet, Parkinson's tells me that there is limited time left to take care of any unfinished business. Parkinson's tells me that the finish line is not far off.

Some say they don't need Parkinson's to tell them they are approaching the finish line. They say they understand that life does not go on forever.

I think, however, that there is a big difference between understanding intellectually that life does not go on forever and actually making decisions based on that understanding. Time is a precious commodity. It is one thing to decide how, and with whom, I will spend my time when I think I have a virtually limitless supply of time. It is quite another to make these decisions when I recognize that my time is running out.

The less time I think I have, the more precious time seems. The more precious time seems, the more thought I give to how, and with whom, I spend it.

As mentioned earlier, some recent studies indicate that the average life expectancy of a Parkinson's patient is about the same as the average life expectancy of other people of the same age. Other studies indicate that the average Parkinson's patient lives from 15 to 25 years following diagnosis. Some would point to these studies and say that the Parkinson's bell rings too soon to be useful—that it rings long before time really starts to run out.

I disagree. A bell that rings too soon does me no harm. If the alternative is a bell that rings too late or not at all, I'll take the bell that rings too soon. I am fortunate to hear the bell ring when there is still time to react to it.

I am fortunate in other respects as well. I am more fortunate than other Parkinson's patients whose current symptoms are more severe than mine are right now. I am more fortunate than others with diseases and disabilities far more debilitating than Parkinson's.

Although I sometimes start to feel guilty about my good fortune, I dismiss such feelings by asking myself whether those who don't have Parkinson's should feel guilty about their good fortune. I believe firmly that they have no reason to feel guilty. If they—the people who don't have Parkinson's—have no reason for guilt, why should I feel guilty just because my current symptoms are not as severe as they might be?

At the beginning of the book I mentioned that when I was diagnosed with Parkinson's, I mistakenly focused on the "Why me?" question. This is not the only question that has led me astray. Over the years, I have considered other unanswerable questions, such as how or when I will die from Parkinson's. Many say that Parkinson's is not fatal and that Parkinson's patients die *with* Parkinson's, not *from* Parkinson's. If Parkinson's is not fatal, it is pointless to ask how or when I will die from it.

On the other hand, if the disease is fatal, Parkinson's patients are in essentially the same position as people who do not have Parkinson's. People who do not have Parkinson's do not know how or when they will die. My position is no different. Parkinson's progresses slowly. Even if the disease is fatal, there is no assurance that I will die from it. Something else could end my life first.

I find it much more productive to focus on how I will *live* with Parkinson's.

Myths and Misconceptions

THERE ARE MANY common myths and misconceptions about PD. Here are ten of them, together with brief explanations of why they are myths.

1. *Myth or misconception: Only old people have PD.*

   Truth: The average age of a newly diagnosed PD patient is approximately 60. Even if age 60 is considered "old," 60 is just the average age. As many as 15% of newly diagnosed patients are under age 50 at diagnosis, and as many as 10% are age 40 or less.

2. *Myth or misconception: PD is a movement disorder.*

   Truth: PD is only partly a movement disorder. PD has many nonmovement symptoms as well.

3. *Myth or misconception: All PD patients have tremors.*

   Truth: Most PD patients have tremors, but roughly 25% do not.

4. *Myth or misconception: PD causes patients to have dyskinesias.*

   Truth: Dyskinesias are involuntary movements that are triggered by an excessive levodopa effect. It can be difficult to find a dose of levodopa that provides relief from PD symptoms without causing dyskinesias.

5. *Myth or misconception: PD is caused by genetic factors.*

   Truth: Only about 10% of PD cases have been linked to a genetic cause. The cause or causes of the remaining cases are unknown, but experts believe that these cases are caused by a combination of environmental and genetic factors.

6. *Myth or misconception: Not much can be done to help a PD patient.*

   Truth: Medication, surgery, physical exercise, speech therapy, support group participation, and other therapies all help patients to deal with PD's symptoms if not with the underlying disease.

7. *Myth or misconception: DBS surgery should be performed only on patients with advanced PD.*

   Truth: Experts have reported good results from providing DBS to patients in earlier stages of PD.

8. *Myth or misconception: People with PD cannot live independent and productive lives.*

   Truth: The severity and progression of the disease vary from patient to patient. Most patients can live on their own and be as productive as anyone else of the same age.

9. *Myth or misconception: PD is fatal.*

   Truth: Most PD patients die for other reasons. Although PD does not, by itself, cause death, it can result in such diseases as pneumonia, aspiration pneumonia, or heart disease, which do cause death.

10. *Myth or misconception: PD reduces the patient's life expectancy.*

    Truth: Although some experts disagree, PD appears to have no material impact on the patient's life expectancy.

Although levodopa does not cure PD, levodopa reduces the severity of the disease's symptoms and dramatically improves the health and longevity of PD patients. The mortality experience of PD patients after 1967, when the FDA approved the clinical use of levodopa, is substantially better than the mortality experience of PD patients before 1968. In 1967, a PD patient lived, on average, 5 to 15 years from the date of diagnosis. The corresponding figure today is 15 to 25 years.

APPENDIX 2

Interviews

EVEN THOUGH ALL Parkinson's patients are treated as having the same disease, every patient has a different story to tell. In writing this book, I have relied on individual patients and their partners to describe what life with Parkinson's is like for them. I hope that others will benefit from these candid and thoughtful descriptions.

My interviews with Parkinson's patients and their partners were conducted in 2014 and 2015. The interviewees are identified in the table below. About half of the interviewees are members of the support group in which I participate.

I found that the patients and partners whom I asked to interview were eager to participate. They made it clear to me that they wanted to tell their stories to the public—not because they craved publicity, but because they wanted to help others.

After each interview, I asked the person to review my write-up of the interview and to make any appropriate corrections or revisions. This helped to assure the book's accuracy. Although I recorded most of the sessions, I was concerned that I might miss some nuance or point of emphasis or that the interviewee might remember an important point after the interview was over. In addition, because I was a stranger to about half of the interviewees, I thought that telling them in advance that they would have an opportunity to edit my write-ups would help to make them comfortable rather than guarded.

Some interviewees' views were inconsistent with others' or with my own views. I did not attempt to resolve these inconsistencies. In some cases, divergent views are attributable to divergent symptoms. In other cases, it was not clear to me which view was correct or even whether there was a single correct view.

I anticipated that some people might be reluctant to talk about certain highly personal matters, such as sexual dysfunction. To address such concerns, I gave some patients an opportunity to respond anonymously to questions about such matters. In the book, each such response is identified as coming from an anonymous patient.

Most of the interviewees reside in the San Diego, California, and Washington, DC, metropolitan areas. Other interviewees reside in Kalamazoo, Michigan, and Christiansburg, Virginia.

Interviewees

Patient	Year of Birth	Year of Diagnosis	Partner
Larry Baskir	1938	2008	Marna Tucker
Sarah Boyer	1949	2005	John Boyer
Ivan Brown	1962	2013	Trisha Clark
Anne Davis	1949	2000	Steve Pappas
Judy Dodge	1940	1998	None
Joel Havemann	1943	1989	Judy Havemann
Bert King	1948	2001	Susan King
Scott Kragie	1950	2008	Barbara Woodall
Dan Lewis	1944	1993	Vicki Lewis
Chuck Linderman	1947	2005	Wilma Hazen
Shelly London	1938	2013	Marge London
Fred Moonves	1947	2011	None
Cassandra Peters	1955	2002	Denis Peters
Learie Phillip	1948	2000	Cecile Skinner
Phyllis Richman	1939	1999	Bob Burton

Interviewees *(continued)*

Patient	Year of Birth	Year of Diagnosis	Partner
Sandra Ridinger	1941	2003	Jane Collins (Sandra's sister)
Pete Riehm	1944	2009	Maggie Riehm
Glenn Roberts	1947	2000	Kitty Roberts
Michael Rosenbush (deceased 2014)	1937	2009	Bonnie Kramer
Rick Vaughan	1948	2008	Mary Vaughan
John VerSteeg	1943	1991	Lorrie VerSteeg
Chris Whitmer	1960	2007	Terrie Yoshikane Whitmer

Parkinson's Organizations

THE FOLLOWING LIST of organizations should be helpful to Parkinson's patients and their partners. However, the listing of an organization here should not be interpreted as an endorsement of that organization or its publications. Likewise, the listing of an organization should not be construed as an endorsement of this book or its author by that organization.

Organization	Address	Web Site & Telephone
American Academy of Neurology	201 Chicago Ave. Minneapolis, MN 55415	www.aan.com 800-879-1960
American Parkinson Disease Association, Inc.	135 Parkinson Ave. Staten Island, NY 10305	www.apdaparkinson.org 800-223-2732
Brain Resources and Information Network ("BRAIN")	P.O. Box 5801 Bethesda, MD 20824	www.ninds.nih.gov 800-352-9424
Davis Phinney Foundation	4730 Table Mesa Dr. Suite J-200 Boulder, CO 80305	www.davisphinneyfoundation.org 303-733-3340 866-358-0285
European Parkinson's Disease Association	1 Cobden Road Sevenoaks Kent TN13 3UB United Kingdom	www.epda.eu.com

Organization	Address	Web Site & Telephone
International Parkinson and Movement Disorder Society	555 East Wells St. Suite 1100 Milwaukee, WI 53202	www.movementdisorders.org 414-276-2145
The Michael J. Fox Foundation for Parkinson's Research	Grand Central Station P.O. Box 4777 New York, NY 10163-4777	www.michaeljfox.org 800-708-7644
National Parkinson Foundation	200 SE 1st St. Suite 800 Miami, FL 33136	www.parkinson.org 800-473-4636
Northwest Parkinson's Foundation	7525 SE 29th St. Suite 300 Mercer Island, WA 98040	www.nwpf.org 206-748-9481 877-980-7500
The Parkinson Alliance	P.O. Box 308 Kingston, NJ 08528-0308	www.parkinsonalliance.org 609-688-0870 800-579-8440
Parkinson Foundation of the National Capital Area	8830 Cameron St. Suite 201 Silver Spring, MD 20910	www.parkinsonfoundation.org 703-734-1017
Parkinson Study Group	Massachusetts General Hospital MassGeneral Institute for Neurodegenerative Disease 114 16th St., Room 3002 Boston, MA 02129	www.parkinson-study-group.org 585-273-2862 585-275-1642
Parkinson's Disease Foundation	1359 Broadway, Suite 1509 New York, NY 10018	www.pdf.org 212-923-4700 800-457-6676
Summit for Stem Cell	Mission Edge San Diego, Inc. P.O. Box 12319 San Diego CA 92112	www.summitforstemcell.org 858-759-1610
World Parkinson Coalition	1359 Broadway, Suite 1509 New York, NY 10018	www.worldpdcoalition.org 212-923-4700

Drugs Treating PD Movement Symptoms

Generic Name	Brand Name	What Drugs Do	Chief Potential Side Effects	Comments
Levodopa-carbidopa	Parcopa Sinemet	Increase level of dopamine in the brain	Nausea, low blood pressure, restlessness, drowsiness, hallucinations, dystonia, dyskinesias, nightmares	Wearing-off effect. Usually helps most with slow movement and rigidity. Can reduce symptoms but not a cure. Does not replace lost nerve cells or stop progression of PD.
Apomorphine Pramipexole Ropinirole Rotigotine	Apokyn Mirapex Requip Neupro	Mimic dopamine (dopamine agonists)	Many side effects are similar to those of levodopa; also can cause uncontrollable desire to gamble, hypersexuality, or compulsive shopping.	Less effective than levodopa, but works for longer periods of time.
Rasagiline Selegiline (deprenyl)	Azilect Eldepryl Zelapar	Inhibit dopamine breakdown (MAO-B inhibitors)	Nausea, orthostatic hypotension, insomnia	Can cause dopamine to accumulate in nerve cells and reduce PD symptoms. Can enhance and prolong response to levodopa and reduce wearing off.
Entacapone Tolcapone	Comtan Tasmar	Inhibit dopamine breakdown (COMT inhibitors)	Diarrhea, nausea, sleep disturbances, dizziness, abdominal pain, hallucinations; rarely, severe liver disease	Can prolong effect of levodopa and reduce duration of levodopa's off periods.

Generic Name	Brand Name	What Drugs Do	Chief Potential Side Effects	Comments
Benztropine Ethopropazine Trihexyphenidyl	Cogentin Parsidol Artane	Decrease the action of acetylcholine (anticholinergics)	Dry mouth, constipation, urinary retention, hallucinations, memory loss. blurred vision, confusion	Can be particularly effective for tremor.
Amantadine	Symmetrel	Unknown mechanism of action	Insomnia, mottled skin, edema, agitation, hallucinations	Can reduce PD symptoms and levodopa-induced dyskinesias. After several months, effectiveness wears off in up to half of patients.

Source: National Institute of Neurological Disorders and Stroke, National Institutes of Health, "Parkinson's Disease: Hope Through Research," www.ninds.nih.gov/disorders/parkinsons_disease/detail_parkinsons_disease.htm#3159_11.

My Guidelines

IN COMBATING PARKINSON'S, I follow the guidelines set forth below. I emphasize that these are *my* guidelines; they are not necessarily appropriate for other Parkinson's patients. I hope, though, that they are useful as an exemple.

1. *Consult experts.* Consult a neurologist with expertise and experience in treating Parkinson's. As and when appropriate, consult other expert professionals, such as neurosurgeons, physical therapists, occupational therapists, speech therapists, psychiatrists, and ophthalmologists.
2. *Educate yourself.* Educate yourself about Parkinson's and keep up with developments. Attend seminars and symposia. Consider new therapies. Keep current.
3. *Participate in treatment decisions.* Do not leave decisions to the experts. Raise questions. Make suggestions.
4. *Exercise.* Treat physical exercise as if it were medicine. Like medicine, exercise is mandatory, not optional.
5. *Be persistent.* Combating Parkinson's requires sustained effort.
6. *Be positive.* Be optimistic. Focus on battling the disease right now rather than wondering how much longer you

can keep it up. Instead of asking "Why me?" ask "Why not me?"

7. *Be realistic.* Excessive optimism can breed disappointment and undermine persistence. Temper optimism with realism.

8. *Socialize.* Do not become a recluse. Welcome, rather than resist, assistance. Participate in a support group. Help others.

9. *Avoid stress.* Reduce or avoid stress.

10. *Sleep.* Regularly get a good night's sleep.

Bibliography

Books

J. Eric Ahlskog, *The Parkinson's Disease Treatment Book*, 2d ed. (Oxford Univ. Press, 2015).

John Argue, *Parkinson's Disease & the Art of Moving* (New Harbinger Publications, 2000).

Jackie Hunt Christensen, *The First Year—Parkinson's Disease: An Essential Guide for the Newly Diagnosed* (Marlowe & Co., 2005).

Joel Havemann, *A Life Shaken: My Encounter with Parkinson's Disease* (Johns Hopkins Univ. Press, 2004).

Abraham Lieberman and Marcia McCall, *100 Questions & Answers About Parkinson Disease* (Jones & Bartlett, 2003).

Michael S. Okun, *Parkinson's Treatment: 10 Secrets to a Happier Life* (CreateSpace, 2013).

Jon Palfreman, *Brain Storms: The Race to Unlock the Mysteries of Parkinson's Disease* (Scientific American/Farrar, Straus & Giroux, 2015).

Sotirios A. Parashos, Rose Wichmann, and Todd Melby, *Navigating Life with Parkinson Disease* (Oxford Univ. Press, 2013).

Shelley Peterman Schwarz, *Parkinson's Disease: 300 Tips for Making Life Easier*, 2d ed. (Demos Medical Publishing, 2006).

Nutan Sharma and Elaine Richman, *Parkinson's Disease and the Family: A New Guide* (Harvard Univ. Press, 2005).

Joanne Levin Vine, *I'm Still Standing* (Nortex Press, 2007).

William J. Weiner, Lisa M. Shulman, and Anthony E. Lang, *Parkinson's Disease: A Complete Guide for Patients and Families*, 3d ed. (Johns Hopkins Univ. Press, 2013).

144   BIBLIOGRAPHY

NINDS Reports

National Institute of Neurological Disorders and Stroke, National Institutes of Health, "Parkinson's Disease: Hope Through Research,"
http://www.ninds.nih.gov/disorders/parkinsons_disease/detail_
parkinsons_disease.htm.
National Institute of Neurological Disorders and Stroke, National Institutes of Health, "NINDS Deep Brain Stimulation for Parkinson's
Disease Information Page," http://www.ninds.nih.gov/disorders/
deep_brain_stimulation/deep_brain_stimulation.htm.

Other Publications

Julia Berenson et al., "Achieving Better Quality of Care for Low-Income
Populations: The Roles of Health Insurance and the Medi-
cal Home in Reducing Health Inequities," The Commonwealth
Fund, Issue Brief (May 2012), http://www.commonwealthfund.
org/~/media/files/publications/issue-brief/2012/may/1600_
berenson_achieving_better_quality_care_low_income_v2.pdf.
Andrés M. Bratt-Leal and Jeanne F. Loring, "Stem Cells for Parkinson's
Disease," *Translational Neuroscience* (March 9, 2016), http://
link.springer.com/chapter/10.1007/978-1-4899-7654-3_11.
Jeff M. Bronstein et al., "Deep Brain Stimulation for Parkinson Disease:
An Expert Consensus and Review of Key Issues," *Neurological
Review* (Feb. 2011), http://archneur.jamanetwork.com/article.
aspx?articleid=802237.
Nyshka Chandran, "Harvard-Singapore Team Unveil Potential Parkin-
son's Cure," CNBC, http://www.cnbc.com/2015/07/15/potential-
parkinsons-cure-unveiled.html.
Kendra Cherry, "How Many Neurons Are in the Brain?" *verywell*
(March 11, 2016), https://www.verywell.com/how-many-
neurons-are-in-the-brain-2794889.
B. D. Colen, "Possible Progress Against Parkinson's," *Harvard Gazette*
(March 3, 2015), http://news.harvard.edu/gazette/story/2015/03/
possible-progress-against-parkinsons.
Susan Conova, "Researchers Pinpoint Possible Cause of Familial Forms
of Parkinson's," *In Vivo* 3:10 (Sept. 2004), Columbia University
Medical Center, www.cumc.columbia.edu/publications/in-vivo/
Vol3_Iss10_sept_04/parkinsons_disease.html.
"A Consensus on the Brain Training Industry from the Scientific Com-
munity," Statement of 69 scholars, issued by the Max Planck
Institute for Human Development and the Stanford Center
on Longevity (Oct. 20, 2014), http://longevity3.stanford.edu/

blog/2014/10/15/the-consensus-on-the-brain-training-industry-from-the-scientific-community/.

Ruth-Mary deSouza et al., "Timing of Deep Brain Stimulation in Parkinson Disease: A Need for Reappraisal?" *Annals of Neurology* 73:5 (May 2013), 565–575, http://www.onlinelibrary.wiley.com/doi/10.1002/ana.23890/full.

Rachel Dolhun, "Gut Check on Parkinson's: New Findings on Bacteria Levels," Foxfeed Blog (Dec. 8, 2014), http://www.michaeljfox.org/foundation/news-detail.php?gut-check-on-parkinson-new-findings-on-bacteria-levels.

Cristina Fresquez, "Health Care Barriers Hinder Parkinson's Care for Latinos," Northwest Parkinson's Foundation (June 10, 2013), https://nwpf.org/stay-informed/news/2013/06/health-care-barriers-hinder-parkinsons-care-for-latinos/.

Ellen Garrison, "Non-contact Boxing Aims to Counter Parkinson's Symptoms," *The Washington Times* (Aug. 2, 2015), http://www.washingtontimes.com/news/2015/aug/2/non-contact-boxing-aims-to-counter-parkinsons-symp/?page=all.

Michal Gostkowski, "Parkinson's Disease Management & Treatment Options" (Oct. 4, 2011), Cleveland Clinic, http://my.clevelandclinic.org/health/transcripts/1266_parkinson-s-disease.

Jessica Hamzelou, "Drug Reverses Parkinson's," *New Scientist* 8 (Oct. 24–30, 2015), https://www.newscientist.com/article/mg22830443-900-people-with-parkinsons-walk-again-after-promising-drug-trial/.

J. Patrick Hemming et al., "Racial and Socioeconomic Disparities in Parkinsonism," *Archives of Neurology* 68:4 (April 2011), 498–503, http://archneur.jamanetwork.com/article.aspx?articleid=802818.

Andrew J. Hughes et al., "The Accuracy of Diagnosis of Parkinsonian Syndromes in a Specialist Movement Disorder Service," *Brain* 125:4 (April 2002), 861–870, https://www.researchgate.net/publication/11452566_The_accuracy_of_diagnosis_of_parkinsonian_syndromes_in_a_specialist_movement_disorder_service_Brain.

Johns Hopkins Medicine, "What is Parkinson's Disease?" http://www.hopkinsmedicine.org/neurology_neurosurgery/centers_clinics/movement_disorders/conditions/parkinsons_disease.html.

Michael Kinsley, "Have You Lost Your Mind?" *The New Yorker* (April 28, 2014), http://www.newyorker.com/magazine/2014/04/28/have-you-lost-your-mind.

Andrea K. McDaniels, "Treatment for Parkinson's Could Replace Surgery," *The Baltimore Sun* (Sept. 7, 2015), www.baltimoresun.com/health/bs-hs-parkinson-surgery-20150907-story.html.

Nathan Pankratz and Tatiana Foroud, "Genetics of Parkinson Disease," *Genetics in Medicine* 9 (2007), 801–811, http://www.nature.com/gim/journal/v9/n12/full/gim2007120a.html.

Parkinson's Disease Foundation, "Statistics on Parkinson's," http://www.pdf.org/en/parkinson_statistics.

Sara Reardon and David Cyranoski, "Japan Stem-Cell Trial Stirs Envy," *Nature* (Sept. 16, 2014), http://www.nature.com/news/japan-stem-cell-trial-stirs-envy-1.15935.

Phyllis Richman, "Singing Allows People with Parkinson's Disease to Exercise Their Vocal Cords," *Washington Post* (April 2, 2012), http://www.washingtonpost.com/national/health-science/singing-allows-people-with-parkinsons-disease-to-exercise-their-vocal-cords/2012/04/02/gIQADtYMrS_story.html.

Ted L. Rothstein and C. Warren Olanow, "The Neglected Side of Parkinson's Disease," *American Scientist* 96:3 (May–June 2008), 218–225, http://www.americanscientist.org/issues/feature/2008/3/the-neglected-side-of-parkinsons-disease.

Patrick Sweeney, "Parkinson's Disease," Cleveland Clinic Center for Continuing Education, http://www.clevelandclinicmeded.com/medicalpubs/diseasemanagement/neurology/parkinsons-disease/#prevalence.

University of Bath (Press Release), "Sticky Protein Hails New Approach for Treating Parkinson's" (Feb. 25, 2015), http://www.eurekalert.org/pub_releases/2015-02/pu-sph022515.php.

D. M. Wallace et al., "Sleep-Related Falling Out of Bed in Parkinson's Disease," *Journal of Clinical Neurology* 8:1 (March 2012), 51–57, http://www.ncbi.nlm.nih.gov/pmc/articles/PMC3325432/.

Allison W. Willis et al., "Predictors of Survival in Patients with Parkinson Disease," *Archives of Neurology* 69:5 (May 2012), 601–607, http://archneur.jamanetwork.com/article.aspx?articleid=1149703.

Acknowledgments

I HAVE RELIED heavily on the words and views of the Parkinson's patients and partners whom I interviewed: Larry Baskir and Marna Tucker, Sarah and John Boyer, Ivan Brown and Trisha Clark, Anne Davis, Judy Dodge, Joel and Judy Havemann, Bert and Susan King, Scott Kragie and Barbara Woodall, Dan and Vicki Lewis, Chuck Linderman and Wilma Hazen, Shelly and Marge London, Fred Moonves, Cassandra Peters, Learie Phillip, Phyllis Richman and Bob Burton, Sandra Ridinger, Pete and Maggie Riehm, Glenn and Kitty Roberts, Michael Rosenbush and Bonnie Kramer, Rick Vaughan, John and Lorrie VerSteeg, and Chris Whitmer.

They are the heart and soul of this book. I am very grateful to each of them. Although recounting their Parkinson's experiences was not easy, they did so without hesitation or complaint. In their interviews, they displayed qualities that pervade the Parkinson's community: generosity, candor, courage, wisdom, and determination.

The help and encouragement that Dan and Vicki Lewis and Joel and Judy Havemann gave me bear special mention. They offered sound advice, corrected my errors, and encouraged me to finish the book.

The book itself was the idea of Bill Daniel, one of my college roommates and a gifted writer. When I was slow to get started and even slower to produce, Bill was patient, persistent, and positive.

I will always be grateful for the medical and surgical care (and advice) of William Anderson, Stephen Grill, Fred Lenz, Phillip Pulaski, Jim Ramey, and Nancy Thomas. Dr. Grill's thoughtful and detailed comments in particular helped me to avoid numerous errors in this book.

Thanks also to researchers Andrés Bratt-Leal, Sherry Gould, Jeanne Loring, and Fernando Pagan for their generous advice and support.

I cannot give enough thanks to Leslie Kessler and Bob Seymour, my voice and physical therapists. I could not have done this without you.

I am also grateful for the advice and encouragement of Amy Moore, Bruce Brafman, John Buchanan, Jared Cohen, Kate Deal, Andy Friedman, Kathy Grimsby, Joe and Merna Gutentag, Jeff Huvelle, Keith Lieberthal, Jane and Ken Lieberthal, Liza Lutzker, Kendra Roberson, Joan and Stuart Rubin, Diane Sawtelle, Pete Sawyer, Emin Toro, and Kurt Wimmer.

The help of Paul Dry, Doug Gordon, Dermot Mac Cormack, and Susan Thomas was essential to transform a rough draft to a polished, final product. You have my thanks and admiration for your patience, persistence, and professionalism, as well as your attention to detail.

From start to finish, my family provided both the support I needed and more support than I deserved: my wife, Joanne Levin Vine; my sons, David Vine, Adam Vine, Brian Levin, and Todd Levin; my brothers and their wives, Hugh and Lydia Vine and Ed and Ellen Singer-Vine; and other family members, Jeremy Singer-Vine; Sara and Charles Fabrikant; Jeff and Donna Applestein; Lisa and Gideon Blumenthal; Lauren and Aaron Dworkin; and Susan Dworkin. They were constructive critics and generous contributors.

I have sought to make this book as accurate as possible. Any errors are solely my responsibility.

Index